GUIDELINES FOR

PERINATAL CARE

Third Edition

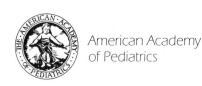

American Academy
of Pediatrics

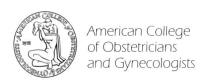

American College
of Obstetricians
and Gynecologists

Supported in part by

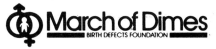

March of Dimes
BIRTH DEFECTS FOUNDATION

Cover and Text Design: Christine Draughn

Guidelines for Perinatal Care was developed through the cooperative efforts of the AAP Committee on Fetus and Newborn and the ACOG Committee on Obstetrics: Maternal and Fetal Medicine. The guidelines should not be viewed as a body of rigid rules. They are general and intended to be adapted to many different situations, taking into account the needs and resources particular to the locality, the institution, or type of practice. Variations and innovations that improve the quality of patient care are to be encouraged rather than restricted. The purpose of these guidelines will be well served if they provide a firm basis on which local norms may be built. The segments related to obstetric practice do not replace the ACOG *Standards for Obstetric–Gynecologic Services*, but rather expand on the principles suggested therein.

Copyright © 1992 by the American Academy of Pediatrics and the American College of Obstetricians and Gynecologists

Library of Congress Cataloging-in-Publication Data
Guidelines for perinatal care.—Third Edition
    p. cm.
    "Developed through the cooperative efforts of the AAP Committee on Fetus and Newborn and the ACOG Committee on Obstetrics: Maternal and Fetal Medicine"—T.p. verso.
    Includes bibliographical references and index.
    ISBN 0-915473-15-1: $40.00
    1. Perinatology—Standards. I. American Academy of Pediatrics. Committee on Fetus and Newborn. II. ACOG Committee on Obstetrics: Maternal and Fetal Medicine.
    [DNLM: 1. Perinatology—standards. WQ 210 G955]
RG600.G85 1992
618.3'2—dc20
DNLM/DLC
for Library of Congress   91-33151
                                                   CIP
ISBN 0-915473-15-1

Quantity prices available on request. Address all orders to AAP; inquiries regarding content may be directed to the respective organizations:

American Academy of Pediatrics
141 Northwest Point Road
PO Box 927
Elk Grove Village, IL 60009-0927

American College of Obstetricians and Gynecologists
409 12th Street, SW
Washington, DC 20024-2188

Editorial Committee

Editors: Roger K. Freeman, MD, FACOG
Ronald L. Poland, MD, FAAP

Associate Editors: John C. Hauth, MD, FACOG
Gerald B. Merenstein, MD, FAAP

ACOG Editorial Staff: Rebecca D. Rinehart
Kathleen E. Achor

Staff: *ACOG*
Harold A. Kaminetzky, MD, FACOG
Shirley A. Shelton
AAP
Mary P. Byas, BSN, MPH
Raymond J. Koteras, MHA
Susan M. Tellez

AAP Committee on Fetus and Newborn

Members,   Gerald B. Merenstein, MD (*Chairman*)
1990–1991   George Cassady, MD
Allen Erenberg, MD
Marilyn Escobedo, MD
Bernard H. Feldman, MD, MPH
Stephen A. Fernbach, MD
Leonard I. Kleinman, MD
Irwin J. Light, MD
William Oh, MD

Liaison Representatives
Alexander Allen, MD
John C. Hauth, MD
Carole Kenner, BSN, MSN, DNS
Linda L. Wright, MD

Past Members,   Ronald L. Poland, MD (*Chairman*)
1988–1990   John W. Freeman, MD
John Kattwinkel, MD

CONTENTS

CHAPTER 3

CHAPTER 4

Appendixes

PREFACE

Pregnancy outcome can most effectively be improved
by integrating the skills and knowledge of multiple disciplines.

—Preface to the first edition,
Guidelines for Perinatal Care

The philosophy of the original *Guidelines for Perinatal Care*, published jointly by the American College of Obstetricians and Gynecologists and the American Academy of Pediatrics in 1983, has continued to guide subsequent editions. The collaboration it exemplified—two disciplines dedicated to the improvement of pregnancy outcome—was an innovation. Today, with the rapid changes, shrinking resources, and new demands facing the health care system, the innovation has become an imperative. The traditional concepts contained in the first edition have, with the third edition, evolved into a cohesive, structured approach to the modern delivery of perinatal care.

The concept of a coordinated, multidisciplinary approach within a regionalized system of perinatal care was introduced in *Toward Improving the Outcome of Pregnancy*, published by the March of Dimes in 1976. This document was based on recommendations from the March of Dimes' Committee on Perinatal Health, which was composed of representatives from AAP, ACOG, and other groups unified by a mutual interest in reducing maternal and infant morbidity and mortality. It defined the principle of regionalized care and, in broad and general terms, illustrated a system of shared responsibility in providing perinatal services. A three-level system was originally proposed, ensuring that all patients would have access to care at an appropriate level, according to need and regardless of financial status. The model was widely accepted and adopted and remains current. At the request of AAP and ACOG, the March of Dimes has reconvened the Committee on Perinatal Health and expanded the multidisciplinary group of experts that will refine and update *Toward Improving the Outcome of Pregnancy*.

The publication of *Toward Improving the Outcome of Pregnancy* created the impetus for further unified efforts by ACOG and AAP to reduce maternal and infant morbidity and mortality. The collaboration of the two groups originally focused on what was to have been a revision of *Standards and Recommendations for Hospital Care of the Newborn, Sixth Edition*, published by AAP in 1977, when regionalized care was still a relatively new concept. The result—the first edition of *Guidelines for Perinatal Care*—was not merely a revision but rather a new joint publication that incorporated, broadened, and replaced its predecessor.

Guidelines for Perinatal Care describes the roles of regions, institutions, and individuals in providing perinatal care. It defines levels of care in terms of facilities, equipment, and personnel, from both an obstetric and pediatric standpoint. The integral parts of a regional program are delineated along with what is expected of all members of such a program in an attempt to clarify and evaluate what constitutes quality health care.

Guidelines for Perinatal Care represents a cross-section of different disciplines within the perinatal community. It is designed for use by all personnel who are involved with the care of pregnant women, their fetuses, and neonates in community programs, hospitals, and medical centers. An intermingling of information of all kinds in varying degrees of detail is necessary to address their collective needs. The result is a unique resource that complements the host of educational documents, listed as a new feature in the appendix, that give more specific information.

In this edition, the concept of levels of care has been retained and reconfigured to focus on functions, taking both physical and human elements into consideration in defining services. With the aid of nursing specialists who participated in the development of this edition, the role of nursing has been elaborated and integrated into all aspects of care. Components of care have been organized into a cohesive framework of personnel and physical facilities. Many areas have been expanded to reflect new and emerging information; for instance, specific recommendations for establishing and using combined units, early discharge criteria for mothers and neonates, advances in hyperbilirubinemia and prenatal diagnosis of genetic disorders, and the management and control of infections.

Much of the new information illustrates the importance of ongoing assessment in the evaluation of services. The ACOG antepartum form is used as a perinatal data base and guide to routine assessments. The collaborative approach is evident in issues addressed for the first time, ranging from new techniques for antepartum fetal surveillance and prevention of preterm labor in obstetrics, to advances in neonatal management and surfactant therapy in pediatrics, to recommendations on nutrition, substance abuse, and federal requirements as they relate to both specialties.

The most current scientific information, professional opinions, and clinical practices have been assembled and reviewed in the formulation of the information in this manual, which is intended to offer guidelines, not strict operating rules. Local circumstances must dictate the way in which these guidelines are best interpreted to meet the needs of a particular hospital, community, or system. For instance, the term "readily available," used to designate acceptable levels of care, should be defined by each institution within the context of its resources and geographic location.

Emphasis has been placed on identifying those areas to be covered by specific, locally defined protocols rather than on promoting rigid recommendations.

The content has undergone rigorous review to ensure accuracy and consistency with the policies of both groups. The guidelines are not meant to be exhaustive, nor do they always agree with those of other organizations; however, they reflect the latest AAP/ACOG recommendations in areas that are subject to constant updating. The text was written, revised, and reviewed by members of the AAP Committee on Fetus and Newborn and the ACOG Committee on Obstetrics: Maternal and Fetal Medicine, and consultants in a variety of specialized areas have contributed to the content. The pioneering efforts of those who developed the previous editions must also be acknowledged. To each and every one of them our sincere appreciation is extended.

Editorial Committee

CHAPTER 1

PERINATAL CARE SERVICES

A regional approach to perinatal care establishes a framework for cooperative efforts to reduce perinatal morbidity and mortality. Regionally coordinated health care systems emphasize professional expertise, consultation, communication, and education for the effective use of resources based on local and individual needs. Outcome is not necessarily influenced by facility or service size. However, the availability of appropriate facilities, equipment, and personnel is essential to the effective management of the small proportion of the perinatal population with the highest risks. The manner in which facilities and personnel are organized can promote efficient use of these resources.

Organization

A comprehensive regional perinatal care system provides patient care, education, evaluation and research, and administration (Appendix A). A system of designating three levels of care has been used, although many variations exist. During the past several years, financial and marketing pressures have encouraged some hospitals to raise their "level designation" for perinatal care services, primarily in regard to patient care activities. This tendency contrasts with the classic concept of regionalization, in which tertiary care centers have the facilities to provide complex patient care and also assume regional responsibilities for transport, outreach education, research, and quality control. Attempts to share responsibilities among hospitals have not been uniformly successful and have resulted in different levels of care for different services at a single hospital. The imbalance in the provision of services traditionally delivered by a regional perinatal center (including patient care, research, and regional education programs) has been due to the fostering of a competitive health care market and the growth of prepaid health care. Another complicating factor is the lack of even distribution of subspecialists in neonatal and maternal–fetal medicine throughout the United States.

Regardless of these changes, the following levels of care relating to inpatient services still pertain. In consideration of the increasing complexity of both inpatient and outpatient perinatal care and emphasis on early and perhaps preconceptional access to perinatal care, outpatient triage of perinatal care assumes greater importance. As used in this chapter, the terms level I care, level II care, and level III care encompass the following functions:

Level I

- Surveillance and care of all patients admitted to the obstetric service, with an established triage system for identifying high-risk patients who should be transferred to a facility that provides level II or level III care prior to delivery
- Proper detection and supportive care of unanticipated maternal–fetal problems that occur during labor and delivery
- Capability to perform cesarean delivery within 30 minutes of the decision to do so
- Availability of blood and fresh-frozen plasma for transfusion
- Anesthesia, radiology, ultrasound, electronic fetal heart rate monitoring, and laboratory services available on a 24-hour basis
- Care of postpartum conditions
- Evaluation of the condition of healthy neonates and continuing care of these neonates until their discharge
- Resuscitation and stabilization of all inborn neonates
- Stabilization of unexpectedly small or sick neonates before transfer to a level II or level III facility
- Consultation and transfer agreement
- Nursery
- Parent–neonate visitation
- Data collection and retrieval

Some level I facilities may provide continuing care for neonates who have relatively minor problems that do not require advanced laboratory, radiologic, or pediatric consultative services. Most level I facilities provide care for convalescing babies who have been returned from level II and level III facilities.

Level II

- Performance of level I services
- Management of high-risk mothers and fetuses admitted and transferred
- Management of small, sick neonates with a moderate degree of illness that are admitted or transferred

Some level II hospitals also have intensive care facilities. Most frequently, level II care pertains to the neonatal expertise required to manage otherwise normal newborns weighing between 1,500–2,500 g and in relatively healthy parturients. These situations usually occur as a result of either preterm labor or preterm amnion rupture, or as a result of a relatively mild pregnancy complication such as mild pregnancy-induced hypertension or preeclampsia, idiopathic intrauterine growth retardation with oligohydramnios, or placenta previa. Thus, in these situations, when the estimated fetal weight is 1,500–2,500 g (approximately 32–<36 completed weeks of gestational age), the needed subspecialty expertise is almost always neonatal medicine and not maternal–fetal medicine. Appropriately trained obstetric specialists can and usually should manage these perinatal situations in conjunction with the appropriate pediatrician or neonatal specialist.

Level III

- Provision of comprehensive perinatal care services for mothers and neonates of all risk categories admitted and transferred
- Research and educational support
- Compilation, analysis, and evaluation of regional data
- Initial evaluation of new high-risk technologies

The services needed at a level III facility vary markedly from those at a level II facility. Level III care for newborns weighing less than 1,500 g or under 32 weeks of gestation always requires neonatal medicine expertise and frequently requires that of maternal–fetal medicine. Moreover, in contrast to level II functions, any fetus that may require immediate sophisticated care, such as those with severe immune or nonimmune hydrops fetalis, or fetal anomalies including congenital heart disease, open neural tube defects, abdominal wall defects, or diaphragmatic hernias, should be delivered at a comprehensive level III care center. Frequently, when level III maternal care is needed, the neonate needs no more than level II neonatal expertise. Instances in which maternal intensive care may be needed include severe maternal cardiac or pulmonary disease, severe pregnancy-associated hypertensive conditions (including cardiac, hepatic, hematologic, or renal dysfunction), severe hemoglobinopathies, or active collagen vascular disease.

Personnel

Factors critical to planning and evaluating the quality and level of personnel required to meet patients' needs in perinatal settings include the mission, geographic location, and design of the facility; the patient population; the scope of practice; qualifications of staff; and obligations for education or research. Perinatal care programs at level I, level II, or level III hospitals should be coordinated jointly by medical and nursing directors for obstetric and pediatric services.

Medical Staff

Level I

The perinatal care program at a level I hospital should be coordinated jointly by the chiefs of the obstetric and pediatric services. In hospitals that do not have separate departments of pediatrics and obstetrics, one physician may be given the responsibility for coordinating perinatal care. This administrative approach requires close coordination and unified policy statements. Responsibilities of the coordinator(s) of perinatal care at a level I hospital include policy development, maintenance of standards of care, collaboration with the nursing department, and consultation with staff at those hospitals providing level II and level III care in the region.

A qualified physician or a certified nurse–midwife should attend all deliveries. When certified nurse–midwives are involved in patient care, their specific roles should be delineated by departmental rules and regulations.

Hospitals should ensure the availability of skilled personnel for perinatal emergencies. Anesthesia personnel with credentials to administer obstetric anesthesia should be readily available. At least one person capable of initiating neonatal resuscitation should be present at every delivery. One or two other persons should be available for an emergency resuscitation (see Chapter 3).

Level II

A board-certified obstetrician with special interest, experience, and, in some situations, special-competence certification in maternal–fetal medicine should be chief of the obstetric service at a level II hospital. A board-certified pediatrician with special interest, experience, and, in some situations, subspecialty certification in neonatal medicine should be chief of the newborn care service. These physicians should coordinate the hospital's perinatal care services and, in conjunction with other medical, nursing, and hospital administration staff, develop policies concerning staffing, routine procedures, equipment, and supplies. Small or high-risk neonates should be managed by appropriately qualified physicians. The general pediatrician should have the expertise to assume responsibility for the acute, although less critical, care of the infant; understand the need for proper continuity of care and be capable of providing it; and share responsibility with the neonatologist for the development and delivery of effective services for newborns at risk in the hospital and community. Management may be provided by qualified neonatal nurse practitioners in collaboration with the physician.

The director of obstetric anesthesia services should be board certified and should have training and experience in obstetric anesthesia. Anesthesia personnel with credentials to administer obstetric anesthesia should be readily available. Policies regarding the provision of obstetric anesthesia, including the necessary qualifications of personnel who are to administer anesthesia and their availability for both routine and emergency deliveries, should be developed. The hospital staff should also include a radiologist and, ideally, a clinical pathologist who are available 24 hours a day. Specialized medical and surgical consultation should be readily available.

Level III

Ideally the director of the maternal–fetal medicine service at a level III hospital should be a full-time, board-certified obstetrician with special-competence certification in maternal–fetal medicine. The director of the regional newborn intensive care unit should be a full-time, board-certified pediatrician with subspecialty certification in neonatal medicine. As codirectors of the perinatal service, these physicians are responsible for the maintenance of standards of care, development of the operating budget, evaluation and purchase of equipment, planning and development of in-hospital and outreach educational programs, coordination of these activities, and evaluation of the effectiveness of perinatal care in the region. They should devote their time to patient care services, research, and teaching, and they should coordinate the services provided at their hospital with those provided at level I and level II hospitals in the region.

Other maternal–fetal medicine specialists and neonatologists who practice in the level III facility should have qualifications similar to those of the chief of their service. There should be one neonatologist for every six to ten patients in the continuing care, intermediate care, and intensive care areas. A ratio of one physician (including residents or fellows) or one neonatal nurse practitioner to every four or five patients who require intensive care is ideal for routine daily management. A maternal–fetal medicine specialist and a neonatologist should be readily available for consultation 24 hours a day. Personnel qualified to manage any obstetric or neonatal emergencies should be in house.

Obstetric and neonatal diagnostic imaging, provided by obstetricians or radiologists who have special interest and competence in maternal and neonatal disease and its complications, should be available 24 hours a day. Pediatric subspecialists in cardiology, neurology, hematology, and genetics should be available for consultation. Consultant services in renal function, metabolism, endocrinology, gastroenterology–nutrition, infectious diseases, pulmonary function, immunology, and pharmacology are also needed. In addition, pediatric surgical subspecialists (eg, cardiovascular surgeons; neurosurgeons; and orthopedic, ophthalmologic, urologic, and otolaryngologic surgeons) should be available for consultation and care. Pathologists with special competence in placental, fetal, and neonatal disease should also be members of the level III hospital staff.

A board-certified anesthesiologist with special training or experience in maternal–fetal anesthesia should be in charge of obstetric anesthesia services at a level III hospital. Personnel with credentials to administer obstetric anesthesia should be available in the hospital. Personnel with credentials to administer neonatal and pediatric anesthesia should be available as required.

Nursing Staff

Delivery of safe and effective perinatal nursing care requires appropriately qualified nurses in adequate numbers to meet the needs of each patient in accordance with the care setting. The number of staff and level of skill required are influenced by the scope of nursing practice and degree of nursing responsibilities within an institution. Nursing responsibilities in individual hospitals vary according to the level of care provided, prescribed practice procedures, number of professional and ancillary staff, and professional nursing activities in continuing education and research. Intrapartum care requires the same labor-intensiveness and expertise as any other intensive care unit and, accordingly, should be allocated adequate training and fiscal support.

Changing trends in medical management and technologic advances influence and may increase the nursing workload. Each hospital should determine the scope of nursing practice for each nursing unit and specialty department. A multidisciplinary committee that is composed of representatives from hospital, medical, and nursing administration should follow published professional standards and guidelines, consult state nurse practice acts, identify the types and numbers of procedures performed on each unit, delineate direct and indirect nursing care activities performed, and identify activities that are performed by non-nursing personnel.

Recommended nurse/patient ratios for perinatal services are shown in Table 1-1. Additional personnel are necessary for indirect patient care activities. Close evaluation of all factors involved in a specific case is essential in establishing an acceptable nurse/patient ratio. Variables such as type of patient, patient turnover, acuity of patients' conditions, patient or parent education needs, bereavement care, mixture of skills of the staff, environment, types of delivery, and use of anesthesia must be taken into account in determining appropriate nurse/patient ratios.

Table 1-1. Recommended Nurse/Patient Ratios for Perinatal Care Services

Staffing Ratio	Care Provided
1:1–2	Antepartum testing
1:2	Laboring patients
1:1	Patients in second stage of labor
1:1	Ill patients with complications
1:2	Oxytocin induction or augmentation of labor
1:1	Coverage for initiating epidural anesthesia
1:1	Circulation for cesarean delivery
1:6	Antepartum/postpartum patients without complications
1:2	Postoperative recovery
1:3	Patients with complications, but in stable condition
1:4	Recently born infants and those needing close observation
1:6–8	Newborns needing only routine care
1:3–4	Normal mother–newborn couplet care
1:3–4	Newborns requiring continuing care
1:2–3	Newborns requiring intermediate care
1:1–2	Newborns needing intensive care
1:1	Newborns requiring multisystem support
>1:1	Unstable newborns requiring complex critical care

Level I

The perinatal care program at a level I hospital should be under the direction of a registered nurse. Responsibilities include directing perinatal nursing services, guiding the development and implementation of perinatal policies and procedures, collaborating with the medical staff, and consulting with hospitals providing level II and level III care in the region.

Nursing personnel in each perinatal care area, or combined areas, should be under the direct supervision of a registered nurse. Nursing responsibilities include psychologically and physically preparing the patient and family, applying and monitoring technology, interpreting information and responding appropriately, maintaining an accurate record, and making referrals as necessary. Nursing personnel should be able to identify deviations from normal physiology, especially perinatal emergencies; to institute appropriate actions; and to communicate pathophysiologic processes to primary care providers.

Whenever there are patients in labor in the hospital, the hospital should ensure that a registered nurse is in attendance who has both training and clinical competence in perinatal nursing; can evaluate the condition of the mother, fetus, and neonate; and can assess the degree of risk to which they are subject during labor, delivery, and the neonatal period.

Level II

Each of the obstetric and neonatal patient care areas in level II hospitals should have a head nurse with training and clinical competence in perinatal/neonatal nursing and nursing administration. In addition, specialty certification is highly desirable for all nurse managers, who are responsible for the management of the unit and for supervision of the direct nursing care provided.

In addition to the nursing responsibilities identified under level I hospitals, nursing staff in the labor, delivery, and recovery areas should be especially able to identify and respond to the obstetric and medical complications of pregnancy, labor, and delivery.

Furthermore, the nursing staff of the intermediate care nursery in a level II hospital should be able to monitor and maintain the stability of cardiopulmonary, metabolic, and thermal functions; assist with special procedures, such as lumbar punctures, endotracheal intubation, umbilical vessel catheterization, and exchange transfusion; and perform emergency resuscitation. Nursing staff in this area should be specially trained and able to initiate, modify, or stop treatment when appropriate even if a physician or neonatal nurse practitioner is not present according to established protocols. In those units where neonates receive mechanical ventilation, appropriately trained staff need to be continuously available who have demonstrated the ability to intubate the trachea, manage mechanical ventilation, and decompress a pneumothorax. These activities may be performed by advanced-practice neonatal nurses. The unit's medical director should supervise the delegated medical acts, processes, and procedures performed by advanced-practice neonatal nurses.

Level III

It is highly desirable for the director/supervisor and head nurses of perinatal nursing services in level III hospitals to have not only training and clinical competence in perinatal/neonatal nursing care, but also specialty certification. The obstetric and neonatal patient care areas each should have a head nurse director responsible for management of the unit and supervision of direct patient care. These nurse managers should have at least a nursing baccalaureate degree.

The nursing staff in each perinatal care area, or combined areas, should have specialty certification or advanced training and experience in the nursing management of both low-risk and high-risk patients and their families. Nursing staff should be especially experienced in caring for the obstetric and medical complications of pregnancy or the neonatal period, or both.

The nursing staff in the neonatal intensive care unit should have specialty certification or advanced training and experience in the nursing management of the high-risk neonates and their families. Nursing staff should also be experienced in caring for unstable neonates with multisystem problems and in specialized care technology. An all-professional registered nurse staff is preferable. A clinical nurse specialist should be available for consultation and support to the staff for nursing care issues. Additional nurses with special training are required to fulfill regional center responsibilities, such as outreach and transport (see Chapter 2).

Support Personnel

All Levels

A blood bank technician should always be available for determining blood type, cross-matching blood, and performing Coombs tests. The hospital's infection control personnel should be responsible for surveillance of infections in mothers and neonates, as well as for the development of an appropriate environmental control program (see Chapter 6). A radiologic technician should be readily available 24 hours a day to perform chest X-rays. The need for other support personnel depends on the intensity and level of sophistication of the other support services provided. An organized plan of action, including personnel and equipment, for identification and immediate resuscitation should be established (see "Resuscitation" in Chapter 3).

Levels II and III

The following support personnel should be available to the perinatal care service of level II and level III hospitals:

- At least one full-time medical social worker who has experience with the socioeconomic and psychosocial problems of high-risk mothers and fetuses, sick neonates, and their families (additional medical social workers may be required if the patient load is heavy)
- At least one occupational or physical therapist with neonatal expertise
- At least one registered dietitian/nutritionist who has special training in perinatal nutrition and can plan diets that meet the special needs of high-risk mothers and neonates
- Qualified personnel for support services such as laboratory studies, radiologic studies, and ultrasound examinations (these personnel should be readily available 24 hours a day)
- Respiratory therapists or nurses with special training who can supervise the assisted ventilation of neonates with cardiopulmonary disease (optimally, one therapist is needed for each four neonates who are receiving assisted ventilation)

The hospital's engineering department should include air-conditioning, electronic, and mechanical engineers, as well as biomedical technicians, who are responsible for the safety and reliability of the equipment in all perinatal care areas.

Education

In-Service and Continuing Education

The medical and nursing staffs of any hospital that provides perinatal care at any level should participate in joint in-service sessions on maternal and neonatal care. These sessions should cover the diagnosis and management of perinatal emergencies, as well as the management of routine problems. The staff of each unit should also have a monthly multi-disciplinary conference at which the patient care problems that arose during the previous month are presented and discussed.

The staff of regional centers should assist with the in-service programs of other hospitals in their region on a regular basis. Such assistance should include periodic visits to those hospitals, as well as periodic review of the quality of patient care that those hospitals provide. Regional center staff should be accessible for consultation at all times. The medical and nursing staffs of hospitals that provide level I and level II care should participate in formal courses or conferences sponsored by a regional perinatal resource center. Regularly scheduled regional conferences should include, as a minimum, coverage of the following areas:

- Conferences to review major perinatal illnesses and their treatment and nursing care
- Conferences to review perinatal statistics, the pathology related to all deaths, and significant surgical specimens
- Conferences to review current X-ray films and ultrasound material
- Administrative staff conferences to review procedures and policies
- Teaching seminars for nursing and medical staffs

Perinatal Outreach Education

A program for perinatal outreach education should be designed and coordinated jointly by a neonatal/perinatal physician and a neonatal/perinatal clinical nurse specialist. Their responsibilities should include assessing educational needs, planning curricula, teaching, implementing and evaluating the program, collecting and using perinatal data, providing patient follow-up information to referring community personnel, writing reports, and maintaining informative working relationships with community personnel and outreach team members.

A maternal–fetal medicine specialist, an obstetric nurse, a neonatologist, and a neonatal nurse are the essential members of the perinatal outreach education team. Other professionals (eg, a social worker, a respiratory therapist, or a nutritionist) may also be assigned to the team. Each member should be responsible for teaching, consulting with community professionals as needed, and maintaining communication with the program coordinator and other team members.

Each tertiary care center in a regional system is responsible for organizing an education program tailored to meet the needs of the perinatal health professionals and institutions within the network. Various educational strategies have been found effective, including a series of seminars, audiovisual/media programs, self-instruction booklets, or clinical practicums/rotations. Perinatal outreach education meetings should be held at a routine time and place to promote standardization and continuity of communication among community professionals and regional center personnel.

Physical Facilities

Physical facilities for perinatal care in hospitals should be conducive to care that meets the normal physiologic and psychosocial needs of mothers, neonates, fathers, and families. Special facilities should be available when deviations from the norm require uninterrupted physiologic, biochemical, and clinical observation of patients throughout the perinatal period. Labor, delivery, and newborn care facilities should be located contiguously.

The following recommendations are intended as general guidelines; they should be flexible enough to meet local needs. It is recognized that individual limitations of physical facilities for perinatal care may impede strict adherence to the recommendations. Furthermore, not all hospitals will have all functional units described. Provisions for individual units should be consistent within the framework of a regionalized perinatal care system and the state and local public health regulations.

Obstetric Functional Units

The patient's personal needs and those of her newborn and family should be considered when obstetric service units are planned. The service should be consolidated in one designated area that, ideally, is physically arranged to prohibit nonrelated traffic through the service units. The obstetric service should have facilities for the following functional components:

- Antepartum care for patient stabilization or hospitalization before labor
- Fetal diagnostic testing (eg, nonstress tests, contraction stress tests, amniocentesis, and ultrasound examinations)
- Labor evaluation/observation for patients who are not yet in active labor or who must be observed to determine whether labor has actually begun

- Labor
- Delivery
- Postpartum care

Depending on patient volume and patient care resources available, some of the functional components can be combined in a single room. For example, an admission/examination room may also serve as a labor room or recovery room, or a family waiting room may be used for sibling visitation. To maximize economy and flexibility of staff and space, many hospitals have successfully combined functions into single areas called labor/delivery/recovery (LDR) or labor/delivery/recovery/postpartum (LDRP) rooms. Whether care is provided in a traditional setting, in which separate areas are designated for specific functions, or in a combined setting, all aspects of each component should be retained.

Shown in Tables 1-2 and 1-3 are general guidelines to aid in projecting needs for an obstetric unit. In planning for such facilities, an analysis of the present patterns of care should be reviewed within the context of the following types of information:

- Projected number of births to be served
- The trend in cesarean birth rates at a particular institution
- Occupancy rates that consider "peaks and valleys" in the census
- Present (and projected) number of women in the unit during peak periods, and the length of the peak periods
- The numbers and types of high-risk births
- The anticipated length of stay for women during labor, delivery, and recovery periods

The following facilities should be available to both antepartum and postpartum units and, in appropriate circumstances, may be shared:

- Head nurses' office
- Nurses' station
- Physician and nurse charting area
- Conference room
- Patient education area
- Staff lounge, locker rooms, and on-call sleep rooms
- Examination and treatment room(s)

Table 1-2. Determining Needs of Obstetric Functional Units

Function	Calculation	Comments
	Traditional Setting	
Labor	1 bed (2-bed minimum) for 100–125 annual deliveries	More beds needed if used for other purposes (evaluation, antepartum observation, postpartum recovery).
Delivery	Minimum of 2 rooms (ideally both equipped for cesarean and complicated vaginal deliveries); 2–3 rooms for each 1,000–2,000 annual deliveries	Depends on average number of deliveries per day.
Recovery	One half the number of labor beds	
Postpartum	$\dfrac{\text{Annual deliveries} \times \text{average stay}}{365 \times \text{estimated occupancy rate}}$ = Postpartum beds	Does not allow for antepartum use. Projected 75% occupancy rate lowers risk of patient load exceeding total bed capacity.
	Combined Setting	
LDR	$\dfrac{\text{Annual labor admissions} \times \text{days of stay}}{365 \times \% \text{ occupancy}}$ = LDR rooms	
Postpartum	$\dfrac{\text{Annual deliveries} \times \text{days of stay}}{365 \times \% \text{ occupancy}}$ = Postpartum beds	Certain patients may not use the rooms in some settings (ie, elective cesarean birth or antepartum care). If rooms are not used for a particular function, patient days should be omitted from the calculation accordingly.
LDRP	$\dfrac{\text{Annual labor admission} \times \text{days of stay}}{365 \times \% \text{ occupancy}}$ = LDRP rooms	
Delivery	2 rooms equipped for cesarean or complicated vaginal delivery	Patients who have complications that require operative delivery can undergo delivery in a cesarean birth room. If over 3,500 deliveries are planned and delivery rooms are used for postpartum or gynecologic surgery, additional units may be needed.
Recovery	1–1.5 x number of delivery rooms	Postanesthesia care unit beds are needed unless such care is provided in LDRP.

- Secure area for storage of medications
- Instrument cleanup area
- Area and equipment for bedpan cleansing
- Sitz bath facilities
- Kitchen and pantry
- Workroom and storage area
- Sibling visiting area

Equipment and supplies that should be available include the following items:

- Sterilization equipment (if there is no central sterilization equipment)
- Real-time ultrasound equipment
- X-ray view boxes
- Stretchers with side rails
- Equipment for pelvic examinations
- Sphygmomanometers and stethoscopes
- Fetoscopes
- Fetal monitoring equipment
- Supplies for measuring sugar and protein in urine
- Needles and syringes
- Solutions and equipment for the parenteral administration of fluids

Table 1-3. Annual Birth Capacity per LDR/LDRP Room*

Occupancy (%)	Average Length of Stay (Days)							
	0.5	1.0	1.5	2.0	2.5	3.0	3.5	4.0
90	657	329	219	164	131	110	94	82
80	584	292	195	146	117	97	83	73
70	511	256	170	128	102	85	73	64
60	438	219	146	110	88	73	63	55
50	365	183	122	91	73	61	52	46
40	292	146	97	73	58	49	42	37
30	219	110	73	55	44	37	31	27

*The variable length of stay allows for use of this table to calculate both LDRs and LDRPs.

Hagar DE, Bajok SG, et al. Perspectives in perinatal and pediatric design. Columbus, Ohio: Ross Laboratories, 1988

- Equipment for obtaining blood specimens
- Supplies for analyzing blood gases and determining fetal capillary pH
- Emergency drugs
- Suction apparatus, either a wall outlet or portable equipment
- Urinary catheterization equipment
- Cardiopulmonary resuscitation cart, including:
  — Emergency drugs
  — Needles and syringes
  — Laryngoscope and airways
  — Equipment for delivering positive pressure oxygen
  — Adult cardiac monitor
  — Suction apparatus, if not otherwise provided
  — Defibrillator
- Protection gear for personnel exposed to body fluids
- Ice machine
- Warming cabinets for solutions and blankets

The additional facilities and equipment that are needed for assessing the conditions of the mother and fetus vary with the level of care that the hospital is prepared to provide. Hospitals with a special intensive care section, for example, should have facilities and equipment for the following procedures:

- Comprehensive ultrasound examination
- Fetal monitoring (eg, nonstress and stress testing)
- Maternal monitoring (eg, continuous cardiac and central venous pressure and arterial monitoring)
- Amniocentesis

Patients who have significant medical or obstetric complications should be cared for in a room especially equipped with cardiopulmonary resuscitation equipment and other monitoring equipment necessary for observation and special care. It is preferable that this room be located in the labor and delivery area and meet the physical requirements of any other intensive care room in the hospital. When patients with significant medical or obstetric complications are cared for in the labor and delivery area, the unit should have the same capabilities as an intensive care unit.

Labor

In a traditional setting, a room should be provided for patients in labor. Partitions or curtains are essential to provide privacy in multibed rooms. Each patient should have direct access to toilet and hand-washing facilities, either in or immediately adjacent to each room, which may be shared with an adjoining room. The mother has the option to walk about the room during labor, rest in a comfortable chair, or stay out of bed during the early stages of labor. An early labor lounge is highly desirable.

Areas used for women in labor should be equipped with the following components :

- A labor or birthing bed and a footstool
- A storage area for the patient's clothing and personal belongings
- One or more comfortable chairs
- Adjustable lighting that is pleasant for the patient and adequate for examinations
- An emergency signal and an intercommunication system
- Adequate ventilation and temperature control
- A sphygmomanometer and stethoscope
- Mechanical infusion equipment
- Fetal monitoring equipment
- Oxygen and suction outlets
- Access to at least one shower for use of labor patients
- A writing surface for charting
- Storage facilities for supplies and equipment

The room should have adequate space for support persons, personnel, and equipment. Local regulations concerning the occupancy and size of labor rooms vary; however, single-bed or two-bed rooms require a minimum of 100 ft^2 per bed. Labor rooms used for intensive care of high-risk patients in hospitals that have no designated high-risk unit should be planned with a minimum of 160 ft^2 and have at least two oxygen and two suction outlets.

Delivery

In order to afford easy access and to provide privacy to women in labor, the delivery rooms should be close to the labor rooms. A comfortable waiting area for families should be adjacent to the delivery suite, and restrooms should be nearby.

Traditional delivery rooms and cesarean birth rooms are similar in design to operating rooms. Vaginal deliveries can be performed in either room, whereas cesarean birth rooms are designed especially for that purpose and are thus larger. The traditional delivery room should be 350 ft^2 with a 9-ft ceiling. A cesarean birth room should be 400 ft^2. Each room should be well lighted and environmentally controlled to prevent chilling of mother and neonate. It is desirable that cesarean deliveries be performed in the obstetric unit and that postpartum sterilization capabilities be available there.

Each delivery room should be maintained as a separate unit with equipment and supplies necessary for normal delivery and for the management of complications:

- Delivery/operating table that allows variation in position for delivery
- Instrument table and solution basin stand
- Instruments and equipment for vaginal delivery, repair of lacerations, cesarean delivery, and the management of obstetric emergencies
- Solutions and equipment for the intravenous administration of fluids
- Equipment for administration of all types of anesthesia, including equipment for emergency resuscitation of the mother
- Individual oxygen, air, and suction outlets for mother and neonate
- An emergency call system
- Mirrors for patients to observe the birth
- Wall clock with a second hand
- Equipment for fetal heart rate monitoring
- Neonatal resuscitation/stabilization unit (as defined under "Pediatric Functional Units")
- Scrub sinks with controls strategically placed to allow observation of the patient

Trays containing drugs and equipment necessary for emergency treatment of both mother and neonate should be kept in the delivery room area. Equipment necessary for the treatment of cardiac arrest should also be easily accessible.

A workroom should be available for washing instruments. Instruments should be prepared and sterilized in a separate room; alternatively, these services may be performed in a separate area or by a central supply facility. There should also be a room for the storage and preparation of anesthetic equipment.

Postpartum Care

The postpartum unit should be flexible enough to permit comfortable accommodation of patients when the patient census is at its peak and use of beds for alternate functions when the patient census is low. Ideally, single-occupancy rooms should be provided; however, not more than two patients should share one room. If possible, each room in the postpartum unit should have its own toilet and hand-washing facilities. When this is not possible and it is necessary for patients to use common facilities, patients should be able to reach them without entering a general corridor. When the newborn rooms-in with the mother, the room should have hand-washing facilities, a mobile bassinet unit, and supplies necessary for the care of the newborn. Siblings may visit in the mother's room or in a designated space in the antepartum or postpartum area.

Larger services may have a specific recovery room for postpartum patients with a separate area for high-risk patients. The equipment needed is similar to that needed in any surgical recovery room and includes equipment for monitoring vital signs, suctioning, administering oxygen, and infusing fluids intravenously. Cardiopulmonary resuscitation equipment must be immediately available.

Combined Units (LDR/LDRP)

Comprehensive obstetric and neonatal care can be provided to both the low-risk and the high-risk parturient and infant and their family in a single room. During the labor, delivery, and recovery phases, care can be provided in an LDR room or can be extended to include the postpartum period in an LDRP room. Nurses are cross-trained in antepartum care, labor and delivery, postpartum care, and neonatal care, making the use of staff more cost-effective and increasing the continuity and quality of care. Both LDR and LDRP rooms should be located in or close to the intrapartum area and should be equipped for the same services as those required for separate units.

The LDR and the LDRP rooms are very similar in configuration, with subtle but distinct differences in function. A homelike, family-centered environment with the capability for providing high-risk care is a key design criterion for both the LDR and LDRP rooms. Each room is equipped for all types of delivery except cesarean deliveries or those that may require general anesthesia.

Each LDR or LDRP room is a single-care room with toilet/shower capability and optional tub. A lavatory should be located in each room for the multiple functions of scrubbing, hand-washing, and infant bathing. A window with an outside view is desirable in the LDR and is required in the LDRP, since these rooms are licensed beds. Each room should contain a birthing bed that is comfortable during labor, can be quickly converted to a delivery table, or can be transported to the cesarean delivery room when the need arises. Gas outlets (oxygen, air, and suction) should be provided in two separate locations for the mother and the neonate. Gas outlets and wall-mounted equipment should be easily accessible and may be covered with a sliding surface. Either a ceiling mount or a portable delivery light may be used, depending on the preference of the medical staff.

The zone for the mother should allow space for a sphygmomanometer, stethoscope, fetal monitor, infusion pump, and regional anesthesia administration, as well as resuscitation equipment at the head of the bed. The infant zone should be close to the door, provide three-sided access to the infant, and allow for quick transport to the nursery should the need arise. The family zone should be planned farthest from the entry to the room and should be equipped with a recliner or sofa bed, a rollaway mirror, and a table with chairs.

An enclosed equipment-holding area should be provided in each room and may be shared between two rooms. Ideally, for ease of movement, equipment should be located below the foot of the bed. Standard major equipment held in this area for delivery should include a fetal monitor, delivery case cart, linen hamper, and portable examination lights. A unit equipped for neonatal stabilization and resuscitation, as described under "Pediatric Functional Units," should be available during delivery. In the LDRP, supplies should be included for the postpartum care of the mother and neonate.

The workable size of an LDR or LDRP room is 256 ft^2 with room dimensions of 16 × 16 ft, excluding toilet/shower. This room would be able to accommodate six to eight people comfortably during the childbirth process. A minimum 5-ft clear space at the foot of the bed should be provided for the physician and nurse to occupy during delivery.

Pediatric Functional Units

A pediatric service should have facilities available for the following functional units:

- Resuscitation/stabilization
- Admission/observation
- Newborn nursery
- Continuing care
- Intermediate care
- Intensive care
- Isolation
- Visitation
- Supporting service areas

A region with 25,000 deliveries annually may require 25 beds for intensive care, 75–100 beds for intermediate neonatal care, and 50 beds for continuing neonatal care depending on level of population risk. These beds can be distributed among all the qualified facilities in the region. Frequently, level III facilities within a region also admit maternal and neonatal patients from outside their region. The number of beds needed for these perinatal patients generally must be calculated on the basis of historical referral numbers.

It may be undesirable to establish physically separate neonatal intensive, intermediate, and continuing care areas. For economy of personnel, as well as for primary care nursing, it may be preferable to have a mix of neonatal patients in a single area. Local circumstances should be considered in the design and management of these care areas.

Resuscitation/Stabilization

Immediately after birth, those neonates who require it are resuscitated and stabilized in the resuscitation area. Depending on their condition, neonates are taken from this area to the admission/observation area, the intermediate care area, or the intensive care area in the same hospital, or they are transferred to an intermediate care or intensive care area in a hospital that provides level II or level III care.

The resuscitation area, which should be illuminated to at least 100 foot-candles at the neonate's body surface, should contain the following items:

- Overhead source of radiant heat that can be regulated to the infant's temperature
- Thin resuscitation/examination mattress that allows access on three sides

- Wall clock
- Flat working surface for charting
- Table or flat surface for trays and equipment
- Equipment and medications
- Oxygen, compressed air, and suction sources that are separate from those for the mother
- Heated, temperature-controlled neonatal examination and resuscitation unit
- Equipment for examination, immediate care, and identification of the neonate
- Resuscitation equipment, including laryngoscope, endotracheal tubes, and breathing bags for full-term and preterm neonates

The resuscitation area is usually within the delivery room, although it may be in a designated, contiguous separate room. In the latter case, some institutions have found it helpful to have a window between the delivery room and the resuscitation room through which the neonate can be passed. If resuscitation takes place in the delivery room, the area should be large enough to ensure that the resuscitation of the neonate does not interfere with the care of the mother. Following stabilization of the neonate, if the mother wishes to hold her newborn, a radiant heater or prewarmed blankets should be available to keep the neonate warm. Also, the room temperature should be increased to a level higher than that customary for patient rooms or operating suites. Qualified nursing staff should be available to monitor the newborn during this period.

A resuscitation area should be allotted a minimum of 40 ft^2 of floor space if it is within a delivery room. A separate resuscitation room should have approximately 150 ft^2 of floor space. The area should have adequate suction, oxygen, and compressed air outlets to resuscitate twins and at least six electrical outlets with a capacity of 15 A. A separate resuscitation room should also have an electrical outlet to accommodate a portable X-ray machine, if needed. Electrical outlets should conform to the regulations for areas in which anesthetic agents are administered.

Admission/Observation (Transitional Care Stabilization)

The admission/observation area is for careful evaluation of the neonate's condition during the first 4–24 hours after birth (ie, during the period of physiologic adjustment to extrauterine life). This evaluation may take place within one or more functional areas (eg, the room in which the mother is recovering, the LDRP room, the newborn nursery, or a separate admission/observation area). In some hospitals, the newborn nursery is the primary area for transitional care, both for neonates born within the hospital and for those born outside the hospital. No special or separate isolation facilities are required for neonates born at home or in transit to the hospital.

The admission/observation area should be near or adjacent to the delivery/cesarean birth room. If it is part of the maternal recovery area, which is preferable, physical separation of the mother and newborn during this period can be avoided.

An estimated 40 ft^2 of floor space is needed for each neonate in the admission/observation area. The capacity required depends on the size of the delivery service and the duration of close observation. One patient station is needed for each 150 annual births if the neonate's length of stay in the area is 48 hours. Fewer stations are needed if the neonate's stay in this area is of shorter duration, but there should be at least two stations. The admission/observation area should be well lighted, have a wall clock, and contain emergency resuscitation equipment similar to that in the designated resuscitation area. Outlets should also be similar to those in the resuscitation area.

The physicians' and nurses' assessment of the neonate's condition determines the subsequent level of care. Most neonates are taken from the admission/observation area to the newborn nursery or to the postpartum area for rooming-in. Some neonates require transfer to an intermediate or intensive care area.

Newborn Nursery

Routine care of apparently normal full-term or preterm neonates who weigh more than 2,000 g at birth and have demonstrated successful adaptation to extrauterine life may be provided either in the newborn nursery or in the area where the mother is receiving postpartum care. The nursery should be close to the postpartum area. In a multifloor maternity unit, there should be a newborn nursery on each floor.

The number of bassinets in the newborn nursery should exceed the number of obstetric beds by 25% to accommodate multiple births, extended neonatal hospitalization, and fluctuations in patient load. An additional excess of 10% is appropriate for those hospitals that also have intermediate and intensive care facilities. It is also possible to estimate the required capacity of the newborn nursery on the basis of the mean duration of stay and annual number of liveborn, normal, full-term neonates. For example, if these neonates remain in the hospital an average of

3 days, each bassinet has a capacity of 120 neonates per year (365 divided by 3 = 120). If the average annual number of normal live births is 2,000, an average of 17 bassinets (2,000 divided by 120 = 17) are always in use. Adding 25% of these 17 bassinets to allow for fluctuations in patient census indicates that 21 bassinets are required for this unit. The use of LDRPs and rooming-in decreases this requirement substantially, however.

Because relatively few staff members are needed to provide care in the newborn nursery and because there is no need for bulky equipment, 30 ft^2 of floor space for each neonate should be adequate. There should be at least 3 ft between bassinets in all directions, measured from the edge of one bassinet to the edge of the neighboring bassinet. The newborn care area may be one room in a small hospital or one or more rooms in larger hospitals. Because one nursing staff member is recommended for each 6–8 neonates, individual rooms should have accommodations for 6–8, 12–16, or 18–24 neonates.

The newborn nursery should be well lighted, have a large wall clock, and be equipped for emergency resuscitation. One pair of wall-mounted electrical outlets is recommended for each two neonatal stations; one oxygen outlet, one compressed air outlet, and one suction outlet are recommended for each five or six neonatal stations. Cabinets and counters should be available within the newborn care area for storage of routinely used supplies, such as diapers, formula, and linens. If circumcisions are performed in the nursery, an appropriate table with adequate lighting is required. Electrical outlets to power portable X-ray machines are highly recommended.

Continuing Care

Low-birth-weight neonates who are not sick but require frequent feeding and neonates who require more hours of nursing than do normal neonates should be taken to the continuing care area. This area should be close to the intermediate and intensive care areas so that neonates who have received intermediate or intensive care, but no longer require these levels of care, may be transferred to the continuing care area for convalescence. In level II facilities, this area is also used for convalescing babies who have returned from an outside intensive care unit.

Because the care of neonates in this area requires some bulky equipment (eg, rocking chairs and stools), as well as more personnel than are needed in the newborn nursery, more space is needed per patient unit. There should be 40 ft^2 of floor space for each patient station, with approximately 4 ft between bassinets or incubators.

As in the resuscitation/stabilization and admission/observation areas, equipment for emergency resuscitation is required in the neonatal continuing care area. It may be most conveniently kept on an emergency cart or in a cabinet, but it should be readily available. There should be four electrical outlets, one oxygen outlet, one compressed air outlet, and one suction outlet for each neonatal station. In addition, the equipment and supplies required in the newborn nursery should be available in the continuing care area. Provisions should be made for the comfort of parents or personnel who feed neonates in both incubators and bassinets.

Intermediate Care

Sick neonates who do not require intensive care but require 6–12 hours of nursing time each day should be taken to the intermediate care area. Infants requiring complex care, such as assisted ventilation, for more than several hours should be moved to an intensive care area.

The neonatal intermediate care area should be close to the delivery/cesarean birth room and the intensive care area, and away from general hospital traffic. It should have radiant heaters or incubators for maintaining body temperature, as well as infusion pumps, cardiopulmonary monitors, and equipment for ventilatory assistance.

An estimated 50 ft^2 of floor space is needed for every patient station. Space needed for other purposes (eg, for desks, counters, cabinets, corridors, and treatment rooms) should be added to the space needed for patients. There should be at least 4 ft between incubators, bassinets, or radiant heaters in intermediate care areas. Aisles should be 5 ft wide.

Neonates receiving intermediate care may be housed in a single large room or in two or more smaller rooms. In the latter case, each room should accommodate some multiple of four infant stations, because one nursing staff member is generally required for every three or four neonates who require intermediate care. Large rooms allow greater flexibility in the use of equipment and the assignment of personnel.

Eight electrical outlets, two oxygen outlets, two compressed air outlets, and two suction outlets should be provided for each patient station. In addition, the area should have a special outlet to power the neonatal unit's portable X-ray machine. All electrical outlets for each patient station should be connected to both regular and auxiliary power. An oxygen tank for emergency use should be available for each infant receiving oxygen.

All equipment and supplies for resuscitation should be immediately available within the intermediate care unit. These items may be conveniently placed on an emergency cart.

Intensive Care

Constant nursing and continuous cardiopulmonary and other support for severely ill infants should be provided in the intensive care area. Because emergency care is provided in this area, laboratory and radiologic services should be readily available 24 hours a day. The results of blood gas analysis should be available immediately after sample collection. In many centers, a laboratory adjacent to the intensive care unit provides this service.

The neonatal intensive care area should be near the delivery/cesarean birth room and should be easily accessible from the hospital's ambulance entrance. It should be away from routine hospital traffic. Intensive care may be provided in a single area or in two or more separate rooms.

Not only is the number of nursing, medical, and surgical personnel required in the neonatal intensive care area greater than that required in other perinatal care areas, but also the amount and complexity of equipment required are considerably greater. Therefore, there should be at least 6 ft between incubators or overhead warmers, and aisles should be 8 ft wide. The area should have 80–100 ft^2 of floor space for each neonate, plus space for such things as desks, cabinets, and corridors. In addition, the educational responsibilities of a level III facility require that the design of its neonatal intensive care area include space for instructional activities and office space for data files on the region's perinatal experience.

Each patient station needs 12–16 electrical outlets, 2–4 oxygen outlets, 2–4 compressed air outlets, and 2–4 suction outlets. Like those in the intermediate care area, all electrical outlets for each patient station should be connected to both regular and auxiliary power. In addition, the area should have a special outlet to power the portable X-ray machine housed in the neonatal intensive care unit. An oxygen tank for emergency use should be available for each infant receiving oxygen.

Equipment and supplies in the intensive care area should include all those needed in the resuscitation and intermediate care areas. Immediate availability of emergency oxygen is essential. In addition, equipment for long-term ventilatory support should be provided. Respirators should be equipped with nebulizers or humidifiers with heaters. Continuous on-line monitoring of oxygen concentrations, body temperature, and blood pressure should be available. Supplies should be kept close to the patient station so that nurses are not away from the neonate unnecessarily and may use their time and skills efficiently. A central modular supply system can enhance efficiency.

In some cases, certain surgical procedures (ie, ligation of a patent ductus arteriosus) are performed in an area in or adjacent to the neonatal intensive care unit. Equipment, facilities, and supplies for this area, as well as procedures, must conform to or be comparable to those required for similar procedures in the surgical department of the hospital.

Isolation

Although most neonates with closed-space infections need not be removed from the newborn nursery, provisions should be made for isolating those neonates who may be harboring certain highly contagious agents (eg, varicella, herpes simplex; see Chapter 5). An incubator is not adequate isolation. Because of the inefficiency associated with the use of personnel and space for isolation rooms, neonatal units in smaller hospitals may consider sharing isolation space with another unit of the pediatric service.

Visitation

Parents should have access to their newborns 24 hours a day within all functional units and should be encouraged to participate in the care of their newborns (see Chapter 4). Generally, parents can be with their newborns in the mother's room.

Special provisions may be necessary when neonates are in special care units (ie, continuing, intermediate, or intensive care units). In these situations, mothers are often discharged from the hospital before their newborns and sometimes must travel long distances to be with them. Several systems have been developed to meet the needs of parents and their newborns under these circumstances (eg, rooms for parents in the hospital, adjacent facilities outside the hospital provided by the hospital, or other lodgings nearby). A period of mother–newborn rooming-in prior to discharge is highly desirable when special care is needed. In addition, intensive and intermediate care units require special areas appropriately furnished for counseling of parents, breast-feeding mothers, and grieving families.

Supporting Service Areas

Utility Rooms. Both clean and soiled utility rooms are needed in neonatal care areas. A clean utility room is for preparing formulas, medications, and supplies frequently used in the care of neonates in all functional units. The use of ready-mixed formulas, unit-dose medications, and disposable supplies and equipment has lessened the need for clean utility rooms, however, and they may be replaced by storage areas and clean working surfaces within each functional unit.

A soiled utility room is for storing used and contaminated material before its removal from the care area. This room should contain a counter and a sink with hot and cold running water that is turned on and off by knee or foot controls, soap and paper towel dispensers, and a covered waste receptacle with foot control. A separate deep sink with hot and cold running water should be available for cleaning equipment prior to its return to the central service department for resterilization. Contaminated equipment may be decontaminated in the soiled utility area and transported to the central service department in plastic bags or containers. Contaminated materials should be removed from the care area regularly. Contaminated linen should not be stored in the soiled utility area but should be taken directly from the care area in plastic or other nonporous containers to appropriate hospital facilities.

Storage Areas. A three-level storage system is desirable. The first storage area should be the central supply department of the hospital. The second storage area should be adjacent to or within the patient care areas. In this area, routinely used supplies, such as diapers, formula, linen, cover gowns, charts, and information booklets, may be stored. Generally, space is required in this area only for the amount of each item used between deliveries from the hospital's central supply department (eg, daily or three times weekly). The third area of storage is for items frequently used at the neonate's bedside.

The bedside cabinet storage area should be approximately 8 ft³ for each patient unit in the newborn nursery, 16 ft³ for each patient unit in the intermediate care area, and 24 ft³ for each patient unit in the intensive care area. The newborn nursery requires approximately 3 ft³ per patient for secondary storage of such items as linen and formula. In the resuscitation/stabilization, admission/observation, continuing care, intermediate care, and intensive care areas, there should be approximately 8 ft³ per patient for secondary storage of syringes, needles, intravenous infusion sets, and sterile trays needed in such procedures as umbilical vessel catheterization, lumbar puncture, and thoracotomy.

Large items of equipment (eg, bassinets, warmers, radiant heaters, phototherapy units, and infusion pumps) should be stored in a clean storage area. Approximately 6 ft² of floor space is required for equipment for each patient in the newborn nursery, 18 ft² for each patient in the intermediate care area, and 30 ft² for each patient in the intensive care area.

Treatment Rooms. The development of resuscitation/stabilization, admission/observation, intermediate care, and intensive care areas in which each patient station constitutes a treatment area has largely eliminated the need for a separate treatment room for the performance of procedures such as lumbar punctures, intravenous infusions, venipuncture, and minor surgical procedures. However, if neonates in the newborn nursery, continuing care area, or the postpartum new family unit are to undergo certain procedures (eg, circumcision), a separate treatment area may be necessary. The facilities, outlets, equipment, and supplies should be similar to those of the resuscitation area. The amount of space required depends on the procedures performed.

Scrub Areas. At the entrance to each nursery, there should be a scrub area that can accommodate all personnel entering the area. It should have a sink that is large enough to prevent splashing, with faucets operated by foot or knee controls. Sinks for hand-washing should not be built into counters used for other purposes. The scrub areas should also contain racks, hooks, or lockers for storing clothing and personal items, as well as cabinets for clean gowns, a receptacle for used gowns, and a large wall clock with a sweep second hand for timing hand-washing.

Scrub sinks with foot-operated or knee-operated faucets should be provided for at least every six to eight patient stations in the newborn nursery and for every three to four patient stations in the intermediate or intensive care area. In addition, one scrub sink is needed in the resuscitation/stabilization area, and one is needed for every three to four patient stations in the admission/observation and continuing care areas.

Newborn Bathing Area. Newborns may be given a bath only after their condition has stabilized and they have demonstrated a satisfactory adjustment to extrauterine life. They may be most conveniently bathed in the admission/observation area or in the newborn nursery. The suggested sink size for newborn bathing is $12 \times 24 \times 7$ in. The sink should have knee-operated or foot-operated faucets and a flat surface for drying the neonate. There should be no drafts or forced air vents in this area. Large, prewarmed absorbent towels and an overhead radiant heat source help to keep the infant warm. Scales may be placed in this area so that neonates can be weighed after their bath. Daily baths may consist of sponge baths within the bassinet, as necessary.

Nursing Areas. Space should be provided at the bedside not only for patient care, but also for instructional and charting activities. A flat writing surface (eg, a clipboard) is needed.

A nurses' charting area or desk for tasks such as compiling more detailed records, completing requisitions, and handling specimens may be useful. Physicians may also perform charting and clerical activities in this area. Charting should be considered an unclean procedure, and personnel who have been charting should wash their hands before they have further contact with a neonate.

The head nurse should have an office close to the newborn care areas. Nurses' dressing rooms preferably should be adjacent to the lounge and should contain lockers, storage for clean and soiled scrub attire, toilets, and showers.

Education Areas. A conference room suitable for educational purposes is highly desirable, particularly for level II and level III facilities. It should be in or adjacent to the maternal–newborn areas.

Clerical Areas. The control point for patient care activities is the clerical area. It should be located near the entrance to the neonatal care areas so that personnel can supervise traffic and limit unnecessary entry into these areas. It should have telephones and communication devices that connect to the various neonatal care areas and the delivery suite. In addition, patients' charts, computer terminals, and hospital forms may be located in the clerical area.

Formula Preparation Area. Recommendations regarding the layout, equipment, and procedures necessary for a hospital formula room have been published by the American Dietetic Association. At present, few hospitals prepare their own formulas for the routine feeding of normal newborns, although special formulas may be prepared in formula rooms, diet kitchens, or pharmacies. A recent survey indicated that approximately one half of children's hospitals or hospitals with large pediatric populations had no formula room. Many states have no regulations for the use of formula rooms.

When a hospital does have a formula preparation area, the area should have:

- One to three rooms
- Scrub sink for hand-washing
- Refrigerator dedicated to storage of formula
- Dishwasher
- Adjustable pressure autoclave
- Electronic balance
- Aseptic work area with a laminar flow hood

Such areas can be used for the preparation of infant formulas and enteral formulas for older children and adults. Parenteral nutrition solutions are generally prepared in a separate location.

General Considerations

Illumination. In all newborn care areas, it should be possible to provide approximately 100 ft-c of illumination for the proper evaluation of subtle skin tones and for the performance of delicate procedures. The lighting system should be designed to permit flexibility of illumination and creation of a diurnal light–dark cycle for those infants who do not require constant observation.

Windows. Solid, windowless walls provide the best temperature insulation for neonatal care areas, but they may have a depressing effect on the staff. If there are windows, they should be insulated with double panes. When possible, it may be preferable to use outside walls for non-patient care areas (eg, storage, desks, or charting areas).

Interior Finish. Off-white or pale beige walls minimize distortion of the staff's color perception in patient care areas. This advantage can be nullified by the use of inappropriate fluorescent lighting. Brighter colors may be used elsewhere. Windows in neonatal care areas should have opaque shades that make it possible to darken the area for procedures such as transillumination.

Oxygen and Compressed Air Outlets. Newborn care areas should have oxygen and compressed air piped from a central source at a pressure of 50–60 psi. An alarm system that warns of any critical reduction in line pressure should be installed. Reduction valves and mixers should produce adjustable concentrations of 21–100% oxygen at atmospheric pressure for head hoods and 50–60 psi for mechanical ventilators.

Acoustic Characteristics. The ventilation system, monitors, incubators, suction pumps, mechanical ventilators, and staff produce considerable noise, and the noise level should be monitored intermittently. The construction and redesign for neonatal care areas should include acoustic absorption units or other means to ensure that the sound intensity does not exceed 75 dB and preferably remains below that level (see "Nursery Environment" in Chapter 4). Staff members should take particular care to avoid noise pollution in enclosed patient spaces (eg, incubators).

Electrical Outlets and Electrical Equipment. All electrical outlets should be attached to a common ground. All electrical equipment should be checked for current leakage and grounding adequacy when first introduced into the neonatal care area, after any repair, and periodically while in service. Current leakage allowances, preventive maintenance standards, and equipment quality should meet the standards developed by the Joint Commission on Accreditation of Healthcare Organizations.

At least some (preferably all bedside outlets in intermediate and intensive care areas) electrical outlets should be connected to the hospital's auxiliary power circuit to maintain life support systems in the event of a power failure. The ground on these outlets should be the same as that for the other outlets. Personnel should be thoroughly and repeatedly instructed on the potential electrical hazards within the neonatal care areas.

Safety and Environmental Control. Because of the complexities of environmental control and monitoring, it is necessary for a hospital environmental engineer to ensure that all electrical, lighting, air composition, and temperature systems function properly and safely. The environmental temperature in newborn care areas should be independently adjustable, and control should be sufficient to prevent hot and cold spots, particularly when heat-generating equipment (eg, a radiant warmer) is in use. Humidity should be between 40–60%; it should be controlled through the heating and air-conditioning system of the hospital.

Evacuation Plan

An evacuation policy should be developed for each perinatal care area (ie, antepartum care, labor and delivery, postpartum care, the normal newborn nursery, intermediate care, and intensive care). The policy should specify 1) who orders the evacuation and destination, 2) who designates the assignments, 3) what are the roles and responsibilities of the staff, and 4) what equipment is needed. A floor plan that indicates designated evacuation routes should be posted in a conspicuous place in each unit. The policy and floor plan should be reviewed with the staff at least annually.

Resources and Recommended Reading

American College of Obstetricians and Gynecologists. Standards for obstetric–gynecologic services. 7th ed. Washington, DC: ACOG, 1989

Hager D, Bajo K, Doodan J, Stephens G, Myer S, Smith J. Perspective in perinatal and pediatric design. Columbus, OH: Ross Laboratories, 1988

Jung AL, Streeter NS. Total population estimate of newborn special-care bed needs. Pediatrics 1985;75:993–996

Kattwinkel J. Perinatal outreach education. In: Fanaroff A, Martin R, eds. Behrman's neonatal–perinatal medicine. 4th ed. St Louis: CV Mosby, 1987:16–20

Machol L. LDR: new factor in the OB equation. Contemp Ob Gyn 1988;31(2):176–185

National Association of Neonatal Nurses. Definitions of advanced practice neonatal nursing. Press release, Petaluma, CA: NANN, December 1989

Nurses Association of the American College of Obstetricians and Gynecologists. Considerations for professional nurse staffing in perinatal units. Washington, DC: NAACOG, 1988

Nurses Association of the American College of Obstetricians and Gynecologists. Mother–baby care. Washington, DC: NAACOG, 1989

Nurses Association of the American College of Obstetricians and Gynecologists. Nurse providers of neonatal care: guidelines for educational development and practice. Washington, DC: NAACOG, 1990

Nurses Association of the American College of Obstetricians and Gynecologists. Standards for nursing care of women and newborns. 4th ed. Washington, DC: NAACOG, 1991

CHAPTER 2

INTERHOSPITAL CARE OF THE PERINATAL PATIENT

The transport of pregnant women and neonates between hospitals is recognized as an essential component of modern perinatal care. Regional perinatal care networks should have specific guidelines for the referral of high-risk mothers, as well as sick newborns, to regional centers. There are three types of patient transport:

1. Maternal–fetal transport: Pregnant women are transferred from one facility to another for special care or delivery.
2. Neonatal transport: A team is deployed from one facility to evaluate and stabilize the condition of a neonate at another facility with the intent of transferring the neonate to the team's facility for more intensive care.
3. Return transport: Patients are returned to the facility to which they were originally admitted or to their local hospital for further care when the problems that required transport have been resolved. A return transport is an important benefit to both the individual patient and the system.

The goal of interhospital transport is to care for high-risk perinatal patients in a facility appropriate to their needs. A successful regional referral program is based on a continuum of care that includes the community of origin and involves the following components:

- Risk identification and assessment of problems that will benefit from consultation and transport
- Resource management
- Adequate economic and political support
- Continuous care
- Evaluation and analysis of performance

Indications for Transport

The decision to transfer a perinatal patient should be made by the primary physician in conjunction with a consultant. Both should be well informed about the resources at each perinatal care center because not all centers have facilities for every type of referral. In general, transport should be considered when the resources immediately available to the maternal, fetal, or neonatal patient are not adequate to deal with the patient's actual or anticipated condition. Maternal transport that would benefit the fetus but could seriously jeopardize the mother's well-being should be avoided.

The following conditions require specialized care and may require patient transfer:

I. Maternal conditions
   A. Obstetric complications
      1. Premature rupture of membranes
      2. Premature labor
      3. Severe preeclampsia, eclampsia, or other hypertensive complication
      4. Multiple gestation
      5. Third-trimester bleeding
   B. Medical complications
      1. Serious infections
      2. Severe heart disease
      3. Poorly controlled diabetes mellitus
      4. Thyrotoxicosis
      5. Renal disease with deteriorating function or increased hypertension
      6. Drug overdose
   C. Surgical complications
      1. Trauma requiring intensive care or surgical correction or requiring a procedure that may result in the onset of premature labor
      2. Acute abdominal emergencies
II. Fetal conditions
   A. Anomalies that may require surgery
   B. Rh disease with or without hydrops
III. Neonatal conditions
   A. Gestation less than 32 weeks or weight less than 1,500 g
   B. Persistent respiratory stress
   C. Seizures refractory to usual treatment
   D. Congenital malformations requiring special diagnostic procedures or surgical care

E. Sequelae of hypoxia persisting beyond 2 hours, with evidence of multisystem involvement

F. Cardiac disorders that require special diagnostic procedures or surgery

These examples are to be considered guidelines only; they vary with individual patient needs or institutional capabilities.

Components of Transport

Medical, surgical, and technical advances in perinatal care continue to alter the management of many anomalies and illnesses previously considered lethal. Community physicians should consider seeking help from physicians at their referral center when faced with complex, difficult clinical decisions, especially those decisions involving the use of neonatal life support. Depending on the details of the particular case, consultation may involve either telephone communication or interhospital transfer for further evaluation.

In certain circumstances, the referring physician may manage the transfer personally. Maternal–fetal transports are frequently conducted in this fashion. Transports that originate at the referring hospital, frequently termed one-way transports, function effectively in some locations; however, two-way transport systems, which operate from a base at the center, are more common. Any transport procedure is acceptable if it follows the guidelines given here and attains its goals and objectives.

The provision of adequate life support during the transport of critically ill perinatal patients requires considerable knowledge, skill, experience, and specialized equipment that may not be readily available in all hospitals. Many perinatal care centers that provide level III services have developed two-way transport systems for their service regions because such a regional system provides enough experience to personnel to maintain the skills required for care during transport. Assistance should be sought as soon as the need for transport becomes apparent. This practice reduces the time that the transport team must be in the referring hospital.

Because the demand for tertiary care beds sometimes exceeds the number available, regional centers should have contingency plans. An agreement among centers in neighboring regions that each will accept referrals from the other is probably the most efficient way to resolve this problem. Interunit coordination should be the responsibility of the neonatal/perinatal care staff at each referral center. During periods of high demand, regular communication among the neonatal intensive care units, for example, can provide an up-to-date status report on available beds, preventing a time-consuming, last-minute search and allowing the transport team to focus on a prompt and efficient interhospital transfer.

Informal, poorly organized interhospital care is hazardous. In order to avoid compromising the patient's condition, ensure a predictable response to transport requests, and provide the highest quality of care, the approach to transport should be logical and organized. An interhospital care system has five identifiable components:

1. Organization
2. Communications
3. Personnel
4. Equipment
5. Transport vehicles

Organization

Interhospital care should be available 24 hours a day through a program in which the response time and appropriate capabilities of personnel have been defined. The director of the transport service ideally should be a subspecialist in maternal–fetal medicine or neonatal medicine, or may be a board-certified obstetrician or pediatrician with a special expertise in these subspecialty areas. The director's responsibilities are:

- Quality control of patient care through periodic case review
- Personnel training and supervision
- Development and use of patient care protocols
- Development and use of record-keeping systems and subsequent collation of data for evaluation and analysis
- Regular, periodic review of operational aspects of the program (eg, response times, effectiveness of communications, and equipment maintenance)

Communications

The transfer of a patient from one hospital to another and from one care team to another requires a reliable communications system. It is essential that the referring physician provide the receiving physician with specific clinical information on the patient being referred. The referring physician should carefully evaluate the patient's condition, both in regard to the primary diagnosis and in regard to the development of complicating conditions. Steps should be taken in consultation with staff at the receiving facility to correct these conditions to the extent possible before the transfer.

Maternal patients sometimes require hemodynamic stabilization before transport. It may be necessary to administer tocolytic agents, anticonvulsants, or antihypertensive agents. A patient with cardiorespiratory compromise, active bleeding, rapidly progressive preeclampsia, or rapidly progressive labor should not be transported until her safety can be ensured.

In some situations, maternal transport may not be advisable; neonatal transport may be preferable. If so, the referring physician may arrange for the transport team to arrive at the referring hospital in time to attend the birth. By prior agreement between the referring physician and the dispatch center, the transport team may participate in the initial stabilization of the neonate. While complete stabilization of a newborn is not always possible, transport of an extremely unstable newborn is contraindicated.

Copies of all records, including ultrasound or amniotic fluid studies and fetal heart rate monitoring tracings, should be transferred with the patient. Records may be sent to the receiving hospital by facsimile machine (fax) to be reviewed by the maternal–fetal physician before the patient's transport. A delay in the transfer of the records or failure to transfer them may lead to an unnecessary repetition of studies with concomitant delays in care, increased cost, and risks to both mother and infant.

Complete neonatal and appropriate maternal records should accompany the newborn patient who is being transferred. A tube of the mother's blood should accompany the records. For a neonatal patient, information should be provided that includes details of pregnancy, labor and delivery, physical examination, pertinent initial diagnostic tests, and initial therapeutic interventions. Temporal changes in the baby's condition, in treatments employed, and in responses to treatment should be clearly outlined.

Possession of the appropriate information will enable the receiving facility to prepare for the patient's stabilization, transfer, and admission. Appendixes B and C contain sample record formats for information that can be provided conveniently by telephone. Referral centers in large service areas may establish toll-free lines for referring physicians and families. In metropolitan areas or in small service areas, direct hot lines may link referring obstetric units and nurseries to the perinatal care center.

These lines should be open 24 hours a day and should be well publicized throughout the service region. Communications between the referring and the receiving facilities should include telephone or radio contact during stabilization and transfer.

Dispatching services should provide rapid coordination of vehicles and personnel, as well as communication links between the referring and receiving hospitals and the transfer team. Referring physicians should be given the estimated arrival time of the transport team to ensure the timely availability of appropriate diagnostic studies on which to base therapy during transport. The receiving hospital should also be given an estimated arrival time so that the staff can prepare for the patient's admission. When flights must connect with ground ambulances, it is desirable for a single dispatching center to coordinate the movement of all vehicles.

Personnel

The interhospital care team should have the collective expertise necessary to provide supportive care for a wide variety of emergency conditions in high-risk mothers and neonates. Team members should be drawn from appropriately trained physicians, neonatal nurse clinicians, registered nurses, respiratory therapists, and emergency medical technicians. Composition of the transport team should be at the discretion of the physician responsible for the transport. Transport personnel should be thoroughly familiar with the transport equipment, as any malfunction en route must be handled without the assistance of hospital maintenance staff.

Equipment

The safety and efficiency of a patient transfer are highly dependent on the equipment available to the transport team. The type of transport (maternal or neonatal), the distance of the transfer, the type of transport vehicle(s) used, and the resources available at the referring medical facility determine the kinds and amounts of equipment, drugs, and supplies needed by the transport team.

In the past, many authorities have felt that all transport equipment should be battery operated throughout the transport. In many transport situations, this is still true. However, many ambulances and aircraft are now equipped with converters/inverters that provide 100 V/110 V 400 Hz AC or 24 V/28 V DC power during transport; thus the equipment requires only enough battery power for the portions of the transport that take place outside the vehicles. This arrangement makes it possible to use much less cumbersome, lighter-weight equipment. The integration of multiple modules into the transport vehicle with a single transformer and battery supply greatly reduces space requirements but may lock the transport team into a system that is not easily upgraded.

The equipment needed for transport of a neonate includes an incubator especially designed for transport. It is essential that the transport team be able to monitor the neonate's heart rate, temperature, and blood pressure. An intravenous pump capable of continuous microinfusion is necessary. If ventilator-dependent patients are to be transferred, it should be possible to monitor ventilator pressures and inspired oxygen levels during transport. Devices used to assess blood oxygen levels may be helpful, especially during a long transport.

Equipment for monitoring, resuscitation, and support of both mother and neonate are necessary. In addition, a transport kit that contains essential drugs and special supplies should be available during stabilization and transfer of the patient.

Transport Vehicles

Several factors should be considered in the selection of vehicles for an interhospital transport system. Ground ambulances are adaptable to most short-range transport situations. Fixed-wing aircraft facilitate coverage of a large referral area but are more expensive, require skilled operators and specially trained crews, and may actually prolong the time required for response and transport over relatively short distances because of the time needed to prepare for flight. Helicopters can shorten response and transport time over intermediate distances or in highly congested areas, but they are very expensive to maintain and operate.

The decision to use aircraft in a patient transport system requires special commitments from the director and members of the transport team. During air transport, the pilot should be considered an integral part of the transport team. Therefore, the pilot should be included in appropriate decision-making and should have the authority to change, modify, or cancel the mission for safety reasons. All equipment should be tested to ensure its accuracy and safety in flight. The U.S. Air Force School of Aerospace Medicine maintains records of all medical equipment tested and approved for military aircraft. The American Society for Hospital Based Emergency Air Medical Services, the Aerospace Administration, the Federal Aviation Administration, and the Emergency Care Research Institute can also offer assistance regarding medical equipment suitable for use in aircraft.

Transport Procedure

Medical–Legal Concerns

Many legal details of perinatal transport are not well defined, but all involved parties (eg, the referring hospital and personnel, the receiving hospital and personnel, and commercial ambulance and aircraft charter corporations) assume responsibilities. As spokesperson for the transport team, the referring physician should thoroughly explain the patient's condition and reasons for transfer to the patient or to the parents of the newborn. Informed consent for transfer, admission to the receiving hospital, and care should be obtained. The newborn should be clearly identified.

Federal law places strict requirements on transfers of women in labor by hospitals that receive Medicare funding. Hospitals must be aware of these provisions and make sure that mechanisms for compliance have been established (see Appendix D).

Perinatal transport teams are involved in very special transport situations, and prior attention to potential legal problems is advisable. In most situations, the institution that employs the team is responsible for its actions, and a physician at that institution directs the team's professional activities. Individual hospitals and regions should investigate the use of transfer agreements, which may include the granting of temporary privileges to members of transport teams.

The departure of the transport team from the premises of the referring hospital may be considered the official point of transfer of responsibility from the referring physician to the transport team. Medical–legal responsibility for care of an infant during the stabilization period should be addressed in the formal arrangements between centers. Many hospitals consider patients who are en route and under the care of the transport team to have already been admitted to their institution. Physician–directors and hospital administrators should identify and address the potential administrative or legal problems that may arise in situations in which transport teams cross one or more state lines during a transport. Each institution should establish its own policy.

Interaction at the Referring Hospital

If possible, the referring physician should be at the hospital when the transport team arrives and should remain at the hospital while the team is there in order to ensure complete communication.

The receiving center should receive a report on the patient's condition prior to departure. If the patient being transferred is a newborn, the mother and father should be offered the opportunity to see and touch their neonate before the transfer, even if the neonate is in a transport incubator or on a respirator. An instant picture of the neonate taken prior to transport may be helpful when parents are to be separated from their newborn for some time. The parents should also be given written information about the receiving hospital, including the names of staff members, visiting hours, telephone numbers, and places to stay in the hospital's vicinity. Brochures about the hospital can be useful.

Record-keeping during transport is essential for the continuing care of the patient and for the evaluation of the referral transport process. Records should include the following information:

- Patient's name
- Referring hospital
- Receiving hospital
- Referring physician(s) and telephone number(s)
- Attendants' names and professional status
- Mode of transport
- Time data, including the time of the transport team's arrival at the referring hospital, the time of departure, ground or air ambulance time, and the time of arrival at the receiving hospital
- Patient's age, weight, gestational age, and sex
- Diagnosis and condition
- Procedures performed
- Medication administered
- Periodic vital signs
- Special comments

Patient Care in Transit

A stable patient requires little or no intervention during transport, but should be under continuous observation. The key factors to be monitored in the maternal patient include uterine contractions, cardiopulmonary status, fetal heart rate, deep tendon reflexes, infusion rate of intravenous fluids, and the administration of medications. In the newborn patient, the transport team should frequently monitor temperature, respiration, heart rate, blood pressure, color, activity, and oxygen concentration. A neutral thermal environment should be maintained. It may be necessary to monitor other parameters during transport as well, such as blood glucose levels and blood gases.

The patient, attending personnel, and all equipment should be safely secured inside the transport vehicle. Although it may be necessary to respond rapidly to an emergency, there is seldom need for excessive speed if the patient's condition is stabilized.

Interaction at the Receiving Hospital

The staff of the receiving hospital should be prepared to deal with any unresolved problems or emergencies that involve the transferred patient. Transport personnel should inform the receiving staff of the patient's history and clinical status, as well as all the initial plans for management.

Family members are extremely anxious when a patient is transferred. If they have not been able to accompany or follow the patient, they should be informed of the patient's condition as soon as possible after the patient has arrived. The referring physician and the nursing staff at the referring hospital not only should be informed of the patient's arrival, but also should be kept up to date on the patient's progress throughout the patient's stay at the receiving hospital.

The transfer is not complete until the equipment on the transport vehicle has been restocked and prepared for the next call. Reusable equipment that has come into contact with the transported patient should be appropriately sterilized or decontaminated.

Return Transport

When the receiving hospital no longer provides any unique advantages to those available at the hospital of origin, transport back to the hospital where the mother or infant was originally admitted allows convalescence close to the family members who will be responsible for care after discharge. Furthermore, beds at tertiary care centers are most efficiently used for the most critically ill infants. Return transports are an integral part of a regional transport program.

Outreach Education

Outreach education efforts should reinforce cooperation and coordination of the many skilled persons essential to the interhospital care of high-risk perinatal patients. An often overlooked segment of outreach education is a follow-up report to the referring physician. A prompt and complete report to the referring physician, which describes the patient's condition, the events of transport, and planned therapy, is invaluable. A detailed summary of the patient's condition, which includes recommendations for ongoing care, should be available at discharge. A complete set of medical records is as important in the return transport as it was in the initial transport.

Outreach education related to transport should focus on the following objectives:

- Providers should be informed of the specialized resources available through the perinatal care network.

- Primary physicians should be taught to anticipate complications, to identify high-risk perinatal patients, and to stabilize these patients before transport.

- Quality assurance should be advanced through the continuing education of perinatal tertiary care providers.

- Around-the-clock consultation and referral sources should be established.

Program Evaluation

Regional advisory councils with representatives from the various perinatal care programs can provide a framework for the evaluation of a region's transport system. Such a group can best identify and verify the particular region's needs for interhospital perinatal care. The characteristics of the successful transport system, as described earlier, can be used as a guide for program evaluation. Other criteria should also be considered in evaluating the transport system:

- Availability: Does the system provide all services that may be needed by the perinatal patient?

- Accessibility: Is it possible to connect the patient quickly and appropriately with the services needed? Do those who will need the services know where to get them?

- Responsiveness: Is there a mutual commitment from referring care providers and specialized care providers to honor and accommodate each other's special needs as they arise?

- Effectiveness: Are perinatal patients being given the appropriate care in the appropriate setting? Do physicians and patients regard the perinatal transport service as useful and effective?

As basic as these questions may appear, their answers are often assumed rather than tested. The purpose of an evaluation of the transport system is to collect the evidence about whether or not the system provides high-quality care to high-risk mothers and neonates.

Resources and Recommended Reading

Cowett RM, Coustan DR, Oh W. Effects of maternal transport on admission patterns at a tertiary care center. Am J Obstet Gynecol 1986;154(5):1098–1100

Delaney-Black V, Lubchenco LO, Butterfield LJ, Goldson E, Koops BL, Lazotte DC. Outcome of very low-birth-weight infants: are populations of neonates inherently different after antenatal versus neonatal referral? Am J Obstet Gynecol 1989;160:545–552

Knox GE, Schnitker KA. In-utero transport. Clin Obstet Gynecol 1984;27(1):11–16

Lamont RF, Dunlop PD, Crowley P, Levene MI, Elder MG. Comparative mortality and morbidity of infants transferred in utero or postnatally. J Perinat Med 1983;11(4):200–203

Lubchenco LO, Butterfield LJ, Delaney-Black V, Goldson E, Koops BL, Lazotte DC. Outcome of very low-birth-weight infants: does antepartum versus neonatal referral have a better impact on mortality, morbidity, or long-term outcome? Am J Obstet Gynecol 1989;160:539–545

MacDonald MG, Miller MK. Emergency transport of the perinatal patient. Boston: Little Brown and Co, 1989

Merenstein GB, Pettett G, Woodall J, Hill JM. An analysis of air transport results in the sick newborn II. Antenatal and neonatal referrals. Am J Obstet Gynecol 1977;128(5):520–525

Modanlou HD, Dorchester W, Freeman RK, Rommal C. Perinatal transport to a regional perinatal center in a metropolitan area: maternal versus neonatal transport. Am J Obstet Gynecol 1980;138(8):1157–1164

Paneth N, Kiely JL, Susser M. Age at death used to assess the effect of interhospital transfer of newborns. Pediatrics 1984;73(6):854–861

Paneth N, Kiely JL, Wallenstein S, Susser M. The choice of place of delivery: Effect of hospital level on mortality in all singleton births in New York City. Am J Dis Child 1987;141(1):60–64

Pettett G, Merenstein GB, Battaglia FC, Butterfield LJ, Efird R. An analysis of air transport results in the sick newborn infant: Part I. The transport team. Pediatrics 1975;55(6):774–782

Segal S (ed). Manual for the transport of high-risk newborn infants: principles, policies, equipment, techniques. Ottawa, Ontario: Canadian Paediatric Society, 1972

Sinclair JC, Torrance GW, Boyle MH, Horwood SP, Saigal S, Sackett DL. Evaluation of neonatal intensive-care programs. N Engl J Med 1981;305(9):489–494

CHAPTER 3

ANTEPARTUM AND INTRAPARTUM CARE

A comprehensive perinatal care program involves an integrated approach to medical care and psychosocial support that begins preconceptionally and extends throughout pregnancy and the postpartum period. An important goal of maternal and newborn care is to foster parent–newborn–family relationships. Health care professionals should integrate the concept of family-centered care into every aspect of perinatal services. The process, ideally started preconceptionally, should continue during the first prenatal visit with a review of the parents' attitudes toward the pregnancy, family life, child care practices, stresses in the mother's environment, support systems, and interest in childbirth education classes and be ongoing throughout the perinatal period in both the ambulatory and hospital settings. The active participation of the prospective parents regarding decisions during pregnancy, labor, delivery, and the postpartum period should be encouraged.

Preconception Care

Preconception care can be particularly important in identifying conditions that could benefit from early intervention, such as diabetes mellitus, hypertension, and screening for other metabolic and inherited disorders. For example, the adverse effects of phenylketonuria can be avoided if a special diet is begun before conception and continued throughout pregnancy. Dietary treatment begun after conception is believed to be of less benefit.

When a pregnancy is contemplated, it is desirable for prospective parents to undergo preconception counseling. As a part of a comprehensive examination, information that may have a bearing on a future pregnancy should be obtained. The following components may serve as the basis for a general counseling session:

- Family history
- Genetic history

- Medical history
- Current medication (over the counter and prescribed)
- Substance abuse
- Nutrition
- Environmental factors
- Obstetric history

Antepartum Care

Women who have early and regular prenatal care have healthier babies. Early diagnosis of pregnancy is an important factor in establishing a management plan appropriate for the individual, which should take into consideration the medical, psychosocial, and educational needs of the patient and her family.

Patient Information and Education

The physician and others providing antepartum care should discuss with each patient the type of care that is provided in the office, necessary laboratory studies, the expected course of the pregnancy, signs and symptoms to be reported to the physician (such as rupture of membranes), the timing of subsequent visits, health maintenance, educational programs available, and the options for intrapartum care.

At some time during the prenatal period, communication between the prospective parents and a pediatrician may be helpful. The roles of the various members of the health care team, office policies (including emergency coverage), and alternate physician coverage should also be explained. Specific information regarding costs should be provided. Early in the third trimester, plans for hospital admission, labor, and delivery should be reviewed and information provided on what to do when labor begins, when membranes rupture, or if bleeding occurs.

Analgesic and anesthetic options should be discussed and an attempt made to identify risk factors (see "Analgesia and Anesthesia," this chapter). Because a general anesthetic may be required for emergencies associated with delivery, the patient should be advised of the hazards of ingesting food or fluid after the onset of labor. Aspects of newborn care, including the pros and cons of circumcision of male neonates, should be discussed.

Patients should be provided information about balanced nutrition, as well as ideal caloric intake and weight gain. Patients should be made aware of the benefits of exercise and daily activity and cautioned that a sensation of fatigue suggests that activity has been excessive. Pregnancy is not the time for competitive or dangerous sports or the acquisition of new athletic skills.

Smoking and alcohol consumption should be strongly discouraged. Information regarding cessation programs, where available, should be provided. Patients should be cautioned on the use of drugs, particularly illicit drugs that can have a significantly detrimental effect on the fetus.

A woman with an uncomplicated pregnancy and a normal fetus may continue to work until the onset of labor if her job presents no greater potential hazards than those encountered in normal daily life in the community or home. Most women may return to work several weeks after an uncomplicated delivery. A period of 6 weeks is generally required for a woman's physiologic condition to return to normal, but recommendations regarding the resumption of full activity should be based on the patient's individual circumstances.

Patients should be referred to appropriate educational literature and urged to attend childbirth education classes. Childbirth education classes provide an excellent opportunity for women to obtain specific information about labor, delivery, and postpartum adjustment. Families should be encouraged to participate in childbirth education programs as well. Adequate preparation of family members can have a favorable and lasting effect on the mother, the neonate, and, ultimately, the family unit. Hospitals or community agencies or groups may offer such educational programs. The participation of physicians and hospital obstetric nurses in educational programs is desirable to ensure continuity of care and consistency of instruction.

Serial Surveillance

Antepartum surveillance begins with the first prenatal visit. At this time, the physician or nurse should establish an obstetric data base that contains information regarding the patient's last menstrual period, current pregnancy and past obstetric outcomes, medical and social history, a dietary assessment (see Chapter 7), physical findings, estimated date of delivery (EDD), laboratory tests, and risk assessment. A recommended format for documenting this information is shown in Appendix E. Early identification of medical conditions that can affect pregnancy outcome can minimize maternal and neonatal morbidity by making it possible for the physician to establish an appropriate treatment plan, to maintain close surveillance, and to plan for delivery.

The frequency of follow-up visits should be determined by the individual needs of the woman and the assessment of her risks. Generally, a woman with an uncomplicated pregnancy should be examined approximately every 4 weeks for the first 28 weeks of pregnancy, every 2–3 weeks until 36 weeks of gestation, and weekly thereafter, although flexibility is desirable. Women with medical or obstetric problems may require closer surveillance; the appropriate intervals between visits are determined by the nature and severity of the problems.

At each follow-up visit, the patient should be given an opportunity to ask questions about her pregnancy or comment on changes that she has noted. Blood pressure, weight, uterine size, and heart rate should be assessed during each visit. When a breech presentation is noted at or after 36 weeks, an external cephalic version may be considered. The patient should be asked about fetal movement at each visit after she reports quickening. Urine should be checked to detect protein and glucose. Any change in the pregnancy risk assessment should be recorded after each evaluation and an appropriate management plan outlined. Continual risk assessment should be a standard part of antepartum care.

Tests

Certain laboratory tests should be performed routinely. Additional laboratory evaluations, such as testing for sexually transmitted diseases, testing for genetic disorders, and skin testing for tuberculosis, may be needed based on the history and physical examination. The recommended timing of routine and indicated tests is shown in Table 3-1. The following laboratory tests should be performed as early in pregnancy as possible:

- Hemoglobin or hematocrit measurement
- Urinalysis, including microscopic examination and infection screen
- Blood group and Rh type determinations
- Antibody screen
- Rubella antibody titer measurement
- Syphilis screen
- Cervical cytology
- Hepatitis B virus screen

An unsensitized, Rh-negative patient should have another antibody test at approximately 28 weeks of gestation. If the patient is still unsensitized, she should receive Rho(D) immune globulin prophylactically. In addi-

Table 3-1. Recommended Intervals for Routine Tests and Those Indicated for Individual Patients During Pregnancy

Time (wk)	Assessment
Initial (as early as possible)	Hemoglobin or hematocrit measurement Urinalysis, including microscopic examination and infection screen Blood group and Rh type determinations Antibody screen Rubella antibody titer measurement Syphilis screen Cervical cytology Hepatitis B virus screen
8–18	Ultrasound Amniocentesis Chorionic villus sampling
16–18	Maternal serum alpha-fetoprotein
26–28	Diabetes screening Repeat hemoglobin or hematocrit measurement
28	Repeat antibody test for unsensitized Rh-negative patients Prophylactic administration of Rho(D) immune globulin
32–36	Ultrasound Testing for sexually transmitted disease Repeat hemoglobin or hematocrit measurement

tion, any unsensitized, Rh-negative patient who has an ectopic gestation, undergoes abortion (either spontaneous or induced), or has a condition associated with maternal–fetal hemorrhage (eg, abruptio placentae) should receive Rho(D) immune globulin unless the father is Rh negative.

All patients should be offered maternal serum alpha-fetoprotein testing at 15–20 weeks (ideally at 16–18 weeks). Early in the third trimester the hemoglobin or hematocrit level should be measured again. Repeated tests for sexually transmitted diseases should be performed if the patient is at high risk for these diseases.

Certain risk factors for diabetes mandate maternal glucose screening:

- Family history of diabetes
- Previous macrosomic, malformed, or stillborn infant
- Hypertension

- Glycosuria
- Maternal age 30 years or older

Estimated Date of Delivery

It is of paramount importance in the management of pregnancy to establish an EDD. Problems such as intrauterine growth retardation, premature labor, and postterm pregnancy cannot be managed effectively without accurate information on the EDD. In addition, the gestational age is crucial to the accuracy of certain antepartum tests. If there is a size/date discrepancy, an ultrasound examination is indicated for the purpose of dating. This examination will be most accurate before 20 weeks of gestation.

Accurate dating of pregnancy also relates to the assessment of fetal maturity, which is an important consideration in determining the timing of a repeat cesarean delivery. For patients being considered for elective repeat cesarean deliveries, if one of the following criteria is met, fetal maturity may be assumed and amniocentesis need not be performed:

- Fetal heart tones have been documented for 20 weeks by non-electronic fetoscope or for 30 weeks by Doppler ultrasound.
- Thirty-six weeks have elapsed since a positive serum or urine human chorionic gonadotropin (hCG) pregnancy test performed by a reliable laboratory.
- An ultrasound measurement of the crown–rump length has been obtained between 6–11 weeks that supports a gestational age of 39 weeks or more.
- An ultrasound examination has been performed at 12–20 weeks that confirms a gestational age of 39 weeks or more as determined by clinical history and physical examination.

These criteria are not intended to preclude the use of menstrual dating. If any one criterion confirms gestational age assessment on the basis of menstrual dates in a patient with normal menstrual cycles and no immediate antecedent use of oral contraceptives, it is appropriate to schedule delivery at 39 weeks or later by the menstrual dates. Ultrasound may be considered confirmatory of menstrual dates if there is gestational age agreement within 1 week by crown–rump measurement obtained at 6–11 weeks, or within 10 days by the average of multiple measurements obtained at 12–20 weeks. Another option is to await the onset of spontaneous labor.

Risk Assessment

Identification of risk factors is critical to minimizing maternal and neonatal morbidity and mortality. Although there is a correlation between antenatal risk factors and the development of problems, a significant percentage of problems occur in patients without identified risk factors.

Risk assessment is influenced by medical and obstetric considerations, as well as by the patient's life style and environmental factors. For example, maternal cigarette smoking and low birth weight are known to be related. The chronic, excessive consumption of alcohol during pregnancy is associated with a variety of congenital malformations and other defects. Because the effects of a pregnant woman's moderate intake of alcohol on the fetus and the threshold at which alcohol damages a developing conceptus in a given individual are unknown, it is prudent to avoid alcohol during pregnancy.

Following is a partial list of factors, derived from the history or physical examination, that may increase pregnancy risks and may necessitate further evaluation, consultation, or referral:

Medical Problems

- Cardiovascular, renal, collagen, pulmonary, infectious, hepatic, and sexually transmitted diseases
- Metabolic or endocrine disorders
- Chronic urinary tract infections
- Maternal viral, bacterial, or protozoal infections
- Diabetes mellitus
- Severe anemia
- Isoimmune thrombocytopenia
- Convulsive/neurologic disorders
- Substance abuse (eg, alcohol, tobacco, illicit drugs, prescribed medications [eg, barbiturates, sedatives])
- Nutritional disorders, hyperemesis, anorexia

Obstetric/Genetic Problems

- Poor obstetric history
- Maternal age under 16 or over 35 years
- Previous congenital anomalies
- Multiple gestation
- Isoimmunization

- Intrauterine growth retardation
- Third-trimester bleeding
- Pregnancy-induced hypertension
- Uterine structural anomalies (eg, septum, abnormality caused by in utero exposure to diethylstilbestrol)
- Abnormal amniotic fluid volume (hydramnios, oligohydramnios)
- Fetal cardiac arrhythmias
- Prematurity
- Breech or transverse lie (intrapartum)
- Rupture of membranes for a period of time longer than 24 hours
- Chorioamnionitis

In many instances, special obstetric problems require a multidisciplinary approach to antepartum and intrapartum care. The obstetrician should inform the pediatrician whenever there is a significant risk factor for a neonate. The pediatrician should then meet with the parents and discuss plans for the evaluation and management of the neonate's condition. Some conditions may require transport of the fetus in utero (ie, maternal–fetal transport), which in most circumstances is preferable to transport of the neonate (see Chapter 2).

Genetic Disorders

Couples at increased risk for producing genetically abnormal offspring are usually identified on the basis of advanced maternal age or the presence of a birth defect in the prospective father or mother, their previous offspring, or a near relative. Repetitive spontaneous abortions or stillbirths also constitute grounds for genetic investigation. Certain autosomal recessive diseases are sufficiently common to warrant screening for heterozygosity. For example, such screening should be offered to those of Jewish ancestry to identify carriers of Tay–Sachs disease; to blacks, to identify carriers of sickle cell anemia; and to individuals of Italian, Greek, or Oriental descent, to identify carriers of thalassemia. With the DNA sequence of the cystic fibrosis gene now known, it is anticipated that population screening for this disorder will soon become available; however, at present, routine screening for cystic fibrosis is not recommended. In addition, a family history of autosomal dominant (eg, Huntington disease), autosomal recessive (eg, sickle cell disease), or X-linked disease (eg, hemophilia) is an indication for genetic investigation.

Couples at genetic risk may or may not need formal genetic consultation. Sometimes the problem is relatively uncomplicated; for example, the primary care physician can readily explain the well-known relationship between advanced maternal age and chromosomal abnormalities (Table 3-2). In other cases, complexities may justify referral. Regardless of the

Table 3-2. Chromosome Abnormalities in Liveborns*

Maternal Age	Risk for Down Syndrome	Total Risk for Chromosome Abnormalities†
20	1/1,667	1/526
21	1/1,667	1/526
22	1/1,429	1/500
23	1/1,429	1/500
24	1/1,250	1/476
25	1/1,250	1/476
26	1/1,176	1/476
27	1/1,111	1/455
28	1/1,053	1/435
29	1/1,000	1/417
30	1/952	1/385
31	1/909	1/385
32	1/769	1/322
33	1/602	1/286
34	1/485	1/238
35	1/378	1/192
36	1/289	1/156
37	1/224	1/127
38	1/173	1/102
39	1/136	1/83
40	1/106	1/66
41	1/82	1/53
42	1/63	1/42
43	1/49	1/33
44	1/38	1/26
45	1/30	1/21
46	1/23	1/16
47	1/18	1/13
48	1/14	1/10
49	1/11	1/8

*Because sample size for some intervals is relatively small, 95% confidence limits are sometimes relatively large. Nonetheless, these figures are suitable for genetic counseling.

†47,XXX excluded for ages 20–32 years (data not available).

Modified from the following sources: Hook EB, Cross PK, Schreinemachers DM: Chromosomal abnormality rates at amniocentesis and in liveborn infants. JAMA 249(15):2034–2038, 1983 (ages 33–49); Hook EB: Rates of chromosomal abnormalities at different maternal ages. Obstet Gynecol 58(3):282–285, 1981 indication, counseling is obligatory before antenatal diagnostic studies are performed.

Genetic counseling, whether done by a primary care physician or by a medical geneticist, is a communication process that deals with the occurrence, or the risk of occurrence, of a genetic disorder in a family. In this process, one or more appropriately trained persons attempt to help the individual or family 1) comprehend the medical facts, including the diagnosis, the probable course of the disorder, and the available management; 2) appreciate the way in which heredity contributes to the disorder and the risk of occurrence in specified relatives; 3) understand the options for dealing with the risk of recurrence; 4) choose the course of action that seems appropriate in view of the risk and the family goals, and act in accordance with that decision; and 5) make the best possible adjustment to the disorder in an affected family member and to the risk of recurrence in another family member. The key elements in this definition are diagnosis, communication, and options. When a genetic disorder has been diagnosed in a family member, the counselor should communicate to the family a range of available options; the counselor's function is not to dictate a particular course of action, but to provide information that will allow couples to make an informed decision.

Teratogens

Major birth defects are apparent in about 3% of the general population at birth, although the actual incidence may be greater. An exact cause or mechanism for the defect can be determined in less than 50% of cases. Obstetricians are often asked about potentially teratogenic agents. Although most patient inquiries concern environmental or teratogenic exposure that is related to low-level risks, certain patients will have been exposed to agents that are known to be associated with significant increased risk for fetal malformation and mental retardation. The physician may wish to consult with or refer such a patient to a health professional with special education or experience in teratology and birth defects. Some patients, after they are fully informed of the risks, request pregnancy termination. Whether a woman chooses to terminate or continue the pregnancy, psychologic support for her decision should be provided. Follow-up counseling is also advised for patient education and emotional support after abortion or after the birth of an affected baby. Technical multispecialty support for the liveborn but affected infant is essential.

Many patients raise questions concerning methods for detection. Amniocentesis for chromosome analysis is not appropriate for diagnosis of birth defects caused by teratogens. Ultrasound may detect some structural defects, and open neural tube defects and midline ventral fusion defects may be detected by alpha-fetoprotein (AFP) measurement.

Indications for Testing

The following indications for prenatal diagnostic tests for birth defects have been generally accepted:

- Cytogenetic indications
  - Advanced maternal age (35 years or older at the EDD)
  - Previous offspring with a chromosomal aberration, particularly autosomal trisomy
  - Chromosomal abnormality in either parent, particularly a translocation
  - Need to determine fetal sex when there is a family history of a serious X-linked condition for which specific intrauterine diagnosis is not available
- Single gene disorders (ie, conditions such as inborn errors of metabolism, hemoglobinopathies, cystic fibrosis, and Duchenne muscular dystrophy that are detectable by analysis of chorionic villi, amniotic fluid, or amniotic fluid cells) in a sibling or risk of such disorders because of parents' carrier status
- Multifactorial disorders in a first-degree relative, eg, neural tube defects

Antenatal cytogenetic studies may be appropriate in many other circumstances, depending on the preferences of patients and the availability of scientific expertise. It is unrealistic to expect all primary physicians to be familiar with all genetic advances. Therefore, practitioners should seek consultations with specialists in antenatal diagnosis whenever they are in doubt.

Diagnostic Procedures

The effectiveness of viewing the fetus by ultrasound is well established, and the use of nuclear magnetic resonance imaging for this purpose is under active investigation. Antenatal diagnosis of certain birth defects with these methods is feasible. Ultrasound plays a role in dating pregnancies and excluding multiple gestations whenever antenatal studies are planned. High-resolution ultrasound has been used to diagnose hydrocephalus, neural tube defects, renal abnormalities, skeletal abnormalities, and cardiac anomalies. Expert ultrasonographers have often been able to predict fetal outcomes correctly on the basis of midtrimester studies, although neither the sensitivity nor the specificity of such studies is well defined. Fetoscopic or ultrasound-directed skin biopsies have been used to diagnose certain serious congenital skin disorders of unknown metabolic basis. Percutaneous umbilical cord blood sampling (PUBS) allows recovery of fetal cells and serum useful for detection of genetic disorders and infectious diseases. PUBS may prove reasonably safe. Even though the mortality rate is currently unknown, the benefit may outweigh the risk. One should not perform an invasive test such as PUBS, however, when amniocentesis and amniotic fluid analysis will suffice. The scope of the antenatal detection of genetic disorders has been expanded further by recent rapid advances in molecular biology.

Amniocentesis. Antenatal diagnosis of genetic disorders usually requires fetal cells. Until recently, the only method for obtaining fetal cells was amniocentesis. Transabdominal amniocentesis for genetic purposes usually is performed at 15 weeks of gestation or beyond. An ultrasound examination should be performed prior to amniocentesis to confirm fetal viability, determine fetal age, localize the placenta, and identify multiple gestations. Cytogenetic and biochemical analyses are almost always accurate (99%). Alpha-fetoprotein levels also can be determined on amniotic fluid samples.

Amniocentesis is not without some risk for mother and fetus. Although significant maternal injury rarely occurs, abortion sometimes follows the procedure. The estimated procedurally related risk of spontaneous abortion following amniocentesis at 15 weeks or beyond is 0.5% or less. Injury to the surviving fetus is extremely rare.

Chorionic Villus Sampling (CVS). For diagnosis of genetic disorders in the first trimester, CVS is generally performed between 9–12 gestational (menstrual) weeks. A small sample (5–40 mg) of placental tissue (chorionic villi) is obtained either transcervically or transabdominally. Because villi are fetal in origin, this tissue reflects the fetal genetic status.

Chorionic villi may be analyzed to determine the chromosomal, enzymatic, and DNA status of the fetus. Thus, CVS can be used for the same indications for prenatal diagnosis as genetic midtrimester amniocentesis. However, chorionic villi cannot be used for the prenatal diagnosis of neural tube defects, a diagnosis that requires amniotic fluid AFP. Accordingly, women undergoing CVS should be offered maternal serum AFP

(MSAFP) screening at 15–20 weeks of gestation, optimally at 16–18 weeks.

CVS offers the advantage of first-trimester prenatal diagnosis. The procedure-related risk, however, may be greater than that for amniocentesis. CVS requires appropriate genetic counseling, an operator experienced in performing the technique, and a laboratory experienced in processing the villus specimen and interpreting the results.

Laboratory Studies

Physicians should be aware that many laboratories perform cytogenetic (chromosome) analyses, but relatively few perform certain metabolic tests. Before obtaining specimens, physicians should discuss arrangements with reliable laboratories to ensure that proper preparations have been made to perform the necessary diagnostic studies. This is particularly important in the assessment of AFP to detect neural tube defects (NTDs).

AFP screening during pregnancy has had a major impact on the prenatal detection of fetal abnormalities. Elevated MSAFP levels correlate with an increased risk of NTDs, whereas low MSAFP levels are associated with an increased risk of fetal Down syndrome.

Open NTDs are virtually always associated with elevated levels of amniotic fluid AFP and the presence of acetylcholinesterase, but they are not always associated with elevated levels of MSAFP. Closed NTDs, including those associated with hydrocephalus, are not associated with abnormal AFP findings. Elevated MSAFP levels also exist in multiple pregnancies and certain fetal abnormalities (eg, omphalocele, congenital nephrosis, Turner syndrome with cystic hygroma, fetal bowel obstruction, teratoma). Moreover, small-for-date fetuses and fetal death may be associated with high levels of AFP in amniotic fluid or maternal serum. Incorrect assessment of gestational age may create falsely high or low MSAFP levels.

The laboratory to which MSAFP samples are sent should adhere to a quality assurance program and provide interpretation of results and risk assessment that take into account maternal age, weight, multiple pregnancy, and the presence of insulin-dependent diabetes mellitus. Normative data specific to gestational age (eg, weekly median values) derived from the screened population should be used as the basis for interpretation of results. Relying only on data from a manufacturer's package insert can lead to erroneous interpretation of test results.

Patients with a personal or first-degree family history of NTD should be advised of the risk of having an affected fetus. Because MSAFP screening will detect only 70–80% of open NTDs, these patients should be offered amniocentesis at 15–16 weeks of gestation with amniotic fluid AFP testing. Ultrasound evaluation of the fetus for NTD at 16–18 weeks of gestation can add further information. In patients with no history of NTD (ie, most of the obstetric population), it is now accepted practice to offer the MSAFP screening at 15–20 weeks of gestation. Maximal accuracy requires that the initial sample be obtained at 16–18 weeks of gestation. MSAFP levels are elevated (2.5 multiples of the median [MOM]) in 80–90% of pregnancies in which the fetus has an NTD. Because considerable overlap exists between the MSAFP level in normal pregnancy and the MSAFP level characterized by a fetus with NTD, false-negative and false-positive values are inevitable. Thus, sequential protocols for distinguishing the reason for an elevated MSAFP level other than NTD are needed. Either a second MSAFP test, performed within 1–2 weeks of the time of the first sample, or an ultrasound evaluation without a repeat of the MSAFP test may be performed, depending on the protocol of the laboratory.

Pregnancies with fetal Down syndrome may be associated with low MSAFP levels. A more accurate estimate of the risk of fetal Down syndrome can be made by using a combination of MSAFP level and maternal age. For example, in a 25-year-old woman the risk of delivering an infant with Down syndrome, based on age alone, is 1 in 1,250. If her MSAFP level is 0.36 MOM at 16 weeks of gestation, however, the risk is increased to 1 in 257. The benefit of amniocentesis in such a couple may then outweigh the low yet finite risk of the procedure. When a protocol is used in women under age 35 years, 20–30% of fetuses with Down syndrome can be identified by performing amniocentesis in 2–4% of women. Obstetricians should consult their local provider of genetic diagnostic services concerning the implementation of MSAFP screening and interpretation of results for this purpose. The current practice of offering prenatal diagnosis for the detection of chromosomal abnormalities based on advanced maternal age alone (ie, 35 years or older at the EDD) should continue irrespective of the MSAFP level. In addition to low MSAFP levels, other maternal serum markers proposed to aid in the screening for fetal Down syndrome include elevated levels of hCG and low levels of unconjugated estriol; however, use of these new markers must be regarded as investigational at present.

Antepartum Fetal Surveillance

The primary indication for antepartum tests of fetal well-being is increased risk for uteroplacental insufficiency. A reassuring test result is the usual finding of antepartum tests for fetal well-being and generally justifies a policy of nonintervention in the management of a high-risk pregnancy, barring significant deterioration in maternal condition. Even with persistently reassuring tests, however, perinatal death may occur.

Types of Tests

The two most commonly used biophysical tests are the contraction stress test (CST) and the nonstress test (NST). In a more recently developed test, the biophysical profile (BPP), several different measurements are used to assess fetal well-being. The CST and NST can be performed with standard electronic fetal heart rate monitors, whereas the BPP requires additional ultrasound equipment, as well as clinical expertise, to assess fetal breathing movements, fetal movement, fetal tone, and amniotic fluid volume.

Contraction Stress Test. The CST is based on the fetal heart rate response to uterine contractions. It relies on the premise that fetal oxygenation that is only marginally adequate with the uterus at rest will be transiently worsened by uterine contractions. The resultant intermittent fetal hypoxemia will, in turn, lead to the fetal heart rate pattern of late decelerations. Persistent late decelerations have been shown reliably to reflect suboptimal fetal oxygenation in rhesus monkey fetuses.

The CST is performed with the patient in the semi-Fowler or lateral tilt position, to prevent maternal hypotension and possible decrease in uterine blood flow resulting from the supine position. The fetal heart rate is obtained via an ultrasound transducer, and contraction activity is monitored with a tocodynamometer. A baseline tracing is obtained for 15–20 minutes. If at least three contractions occur in a 10-minute period, no uterine stimulation is necessary. If there are no contractions (or fewer than three every 10 minutes), then contractions can be induced with either nipple stimulation or intravenous administration of low-dose oxytocin.

The results of the CST can be categorized as follows:

- Negative: No late decelerations
- Positive: Late decelerations following 50% or more of contractions
- Suspicious: Intermittent late or variable decelerations
- Unsatisfactory: Fewer than three contractions per 10 minutes or poor-quality tracing

Relative contraindications for CST generally include conditions associated with possible preterm labor, uterine rupture, or uterine bleeding:

- Threatened preterm labor
- Incompetent cervix
- Rupture of membranes
- Vertical uterine scar
- Known placenta previa or suspected chronic abruptio placentae

Nonstress Test. The NST is based on the premise that the heart rate of a normal, healthy fetus will accelerate temporarily with fetal movement. Such heart rate reactivity is thought to be a good indicator of fetal autonomic function; loss of reactivity may reflect metabolic consequences of hypoxemia.

The NST is performed with the patient in the semi-Fowler or lateral tilt position, and the fetal heart rate is monitored with an ultrasound transducer. Preferably, the patient is not fasting and has not recently smoked, as these factors may adversely affect test results. The tracing is observed for fetal heart rate accelerations of at least 15 beats per minute and lasting 15 seconds. If no accelerations occur within a 20-minute period, the tracing is continued for at least 40 minutes to take into account the typical fetal sleep–wake cycle. Some clinicians use vibroacoustic stimulation, which typically will awaken the healthy but sleeping fetus and thereby evoke movement with acceleration.

Results of the NST are considered reactive (negative or normal) if there are two or more fetal heart rate accelerations of at least 15 beats per minute (15 seconds' duration) within a 20-minute period, with or without fetal movement discernible by the mother. A nonreactive tracing is one without acceptable fetal heart rate accelerations over a 40-minute period.

Biophysical Profile. The BPP resembles the NST, as it evaluates the fetus in a resting or nonstressed condition. Unlike the NST, the BPP adds observations obtained from real-time ultrasound to evaluate fetal well-being. The fetus responds to central hypoxemia by alterations in movement, muscle tone, breathing, and heart rate patterns.

The BPP is performed with the patient in the semi-Fowler or lateral tilt position. The patient's bladder does not need to be full during the testing session. A standard real-time ultrasound transducer is placed over the maternal abdomen and the fetus is viewed for approximately 30–60 minutes. The five components are as follows:

1. NST
2. Assessment of fetal breathing movements

3. Assessment of fetal movement (three or more discrete body or limb movements in 30 minutes)

4. Assessment of fetal tone (one or more episodes of extension with return to flexion)

5. Quantitation of amniotic fluid volume

With this method, a score of 2 (normal) or 0 (abnormal) is assigned to each of the five observations. A score of 8 or 10 is reassuring, a score of 6 is equivocal, and a score of 4 or less is abnormal. Even with a reassuring score, oligohydramnios merits further evaluation unless it is due to amnion rupture. Many modifications of the BPP have been reported. The exact independent value of each measurement is not known.

Documentation

Regardless of which antepartum surveillance test is used, a documented, official interpretation should be placed in the patient's chart. If the NST or CST is used, the fetal heart rate tracing, along with a recommended plan for subsequent action, should be noted and maintained. Results of the BPP should be documented. Careful written documentation and timely reporting of test results, especially those of an abnormal test, are essential.

Choice of Test

There is no unanimity of opinion regarding the best biophysical test to evaluate fetal well-being. All three tests (CST, NST, and BPP) have different end points that must be taken into account.

Timing and Frequency

The most important consideration in deciding when to begin antepartum testing is the prognosis for neonatal survival. The severity of maternal disease is another important consideration. In general, with most high-risk pregnancies, testing should begin by 32–34 weeks of gestation. In pregnancies with multiple or severe high-risk conditions, testing might begin as early as 26–28 weeks. A negative CST or normal BPP or a reactive NST in this group is reassuring; however, the significance of abnormal test results is less clear.

When the clinical condition that has prompted testing persists, even though a reassuring test result (reactive NST, negative CST, normal BPP) has been obtained, the test should be repeated periodically until delivery to monitor for continued fetal well-being. The frequency for repeating tests has been arbitrarily set at 7 days, and in general this interval has been accepted. With clinical deterioration of the mother (eg, worsening hypertension, ketoacidosis, hemorrhage), reducing the 7-day interval is prudent. NST or CST tracings showing variable decelerations of at least 15 beats per minute for 15 seconds or longer (as may be seen in the presence of oligohydramnios) may be interpreted as evidence of umbilical cord vulnerability, which should be followed by further evaluation or delivery. Prolonged (1 minute or more) and deep (below 90 beats per minute or 40 beats below baseline) decelerations, regardless of configuration, also may be predictive of fetal compromise and warrant further evaluation.

Prevention of Preterm Labor

Prematurity is the leading cause of perinatal mortality in the United States. Even though there has been an improvement in the survival rate of low-birth-weight neonates, there has been no significant change in the incidence of prematurity over the last 20 years; in fact, rising rates in the United States have been reported.

Achieving a significant decrease in the preterm birth rate may be difficult. Various investigators have reported that preterm premature rupture of membranes initiated preterm delivery in 25–30% of patients and that an indicated preterm delivery for maternal obstetric, medical, or surgical complications accounted for another 20–25%. Thus, at most 50% of preterm deliveries occur in women with spontaneous preterm labor.

Prevention Strategies

Several strategies have been proposed for reducing the rate of preterm labor and birth. Although no strategy has been proved effective, in some populations heightening the patient's and the physician's awareness of the signs and symptoms of preterm labor may help lower the rate of preterm delivery.

Identifying Risk. Following is a list of factors associated with spontaneous preterm labor and birth:

- History of prior preterm birth or midtrimester spontaneous abortion
- Multiple gestation
- Uterine anomaly, including an anomaly caused by exposure to diethylstilbestrol in utero
- Diagnosis of incompetent cervix

- Diagnosed urinary tract infection in the current pregnancy
- Hydramnios
- Second- or third-trimester bleeding
- Diagnosed preterm labor in the current pregnancy
- Preterm premature rupture of membranes in the current pregnancy
- Cervical dilatation of greater than 2 cm in a parous patient and greater than 1 cm in a nullipara
- Low prepregnancy weight (less than 115 lb)

The following complications commonly place a patient at increased risk for indicated preterm delivery:

- Placenta previa or abruptio placentae
- Pregnancy-induced hypertension or preeclampsia
- Chorioamnionitis
- Intrauterine growth retardation
- Certain maternal medical or surgical conditions that exist either before or during gestation

A number of signs and symptoms have been suggested as predictors of preterm labor:

- Frequent uterine contractions (four or more per hour)
- Pelvic pressure
- Increased vaginal discharge
- Diarrhea
- Backache
- Cramping

Educating Providers and Patients About Risks. Studies using historical controls have suggested that provider education regarding high-risk factors and patient teaching regarding the early recognition of premature labor may be effective in preventing preterm birth in some settings. While this approach has been associated with a decrease in the prematurity rate in France, to date none of the published prospective randomized studies in the United States has shown significant benefit in reducing preterm delivery. Nevertheless, it appears reasonable to include risk identification and early recognition of the signs and symptoms of preterm labor as routine components of prenatal care. For those women at high risk for preterm delivery, measures such as increased rest and more frequent prenatal visits may be of benefit.

Establishing Provider-Initiated Contact. Several prospective randomized studies have shown that frequent provider-initiated telephone contact with high-risk patients has been associated with a reduction in preterm birth rates when compared with populations with similar incidences of diagnosed preterm labor. The addition of home uterine activity monitoring to the program has not been shown to add independently to the value of frequent provider-initiated telephone contact. This approach is still under study but, at present, it cannot be recommended routinely. The effectiveness of frequent provider-initiated telephone contact in decreasing preterm birth may result from heightened patient awareness of the early symptoms of preterm labor. Such contact may also decrease the patient's reluctance to contact the provider early, as suggested by findings that preterm labor has been identified earlier in patients in frequent telephone contact groups. This finding may account for the higher success rate reported for tocolysis in women who had frequent provider-initiated telephone contact than that in control patients managed conventionally, even though the control patients were educated in the recognition of the signs and symptoms of preterm labor.

Tocolysis

In some studies, tocolysis of idiopathic preterm labor without maternal or fetal contraindications has been shown to prolong pregnancy, reduce the incidence of preterm birth, and decrease the incidence of low birth weight. In other investigations, despite the efficacy of these agents in delaying delivery for relatively short periods, a reduction in perinatal mortality or in severe neonatal respiratory distress has not been demonstrated. Most clinicians attempt to arrest preterm labor with tocolytic agents at 34 weeks of gestation or less, but approach the management of preterm labor at 34–37 weeks on an individualized basis. Tocolysis may also be of value in preventing delivery during transport to an appropriate facility. The potential risks and benefits of treatment must be weighed against the hazards posed by preterm delivery. The success rates of even appropriately employed tocolysis are limited, however, particularly if the cervix is dilated 3 cm or greater.

Selecting Candidates. The accurate diagnosis of preterm labor and documentation of gestational age are important in the choice of candidates for tocolysis. Tocolytic therapy should be reserved for an overt episode of preterm labor as evidenced by regular uterine contractions persisting after the initiation of rest and hydration and associated with a definite change in cervical effacement or dilatation, or both, preferably documented by the same examiner.

Certain maternal and fetal conditions may contraindicate treatment of preterm labor. For example, severe preeclampsia, chorioamnionitis, and significant hemorrhage usually mandate delivery. In addition, evidence of either acute or chronic fetal compromise may make long-term tocolysis inadvisable. Each case must be judged individually by weighing the suspected risks of continuing the pregnancy versus those of delivery.

Choosing a Tocolytic Protocol. A number of different protocols for tocolysis exist, but a common element of initial management is ensuring adequate maternal hydration. In many patients, preterm uterine contractions will stop spontaneously. Most agents currently used as initial therapy for preterm labor are vasodilators; thus, hydration may have an additional benefit by avoiding a reduction in uterine blood flow secondary to the action of these drugs. Excessive hydration is to be avoided, however, because of the association of pulmonary edema with tocolytic therapy. This usually occurs in the presence of certain risk factors (eg, twins, hydramnios) or in patients receiving tocolytics intravenously for more than 24 hours.

During the initial phase of management, while hydration is taking place, the patient can be carefully evaluated. A history and physical examination and review of obstetric data should help to identify those patients at high risk for adverse effects of tocolysis or of one of the specific tocolytic agents. In addition, this time can be used to estimate the gestational age and to observe the patient for cervical change.

Although the intravenous route has been used in most studies, some practitioners prefer to initiate therapy via the subcutaneous route. Magnesium sulfate and the beta-mimetics ritodrine and terbutaline are the drugs most commonly employed. All three agents have been used successfully in a large number of patients. While all share some risk of maternal pulmonary edema, this risk is greater with beta-mimetic agents. A randomized, controlled comparison of ritodrine and magnesium sulfate demonstrated statistically comparable efficacy and incidence of side effects, although the nature of the side effects of magnesium sulfate was judged to be less serious. Additional advantages of magnesium sulfate are that serum magnesium concentrations are readily available and toxic effects of magnesium sulfate are rarely seen below serum concentrations of 10 mg/dl. Patients in whom contractions continue despite magnesium concentrations of 6–8 mg/dl rarely benefit from higher doses.

Additional tocolytic agents are available, but there are insufficient data on their use in patients to allow recommendation for general use. Antiprostaglandins, such as indomethacin, given orally may provide success comparable to that achieved with intravenous agents, although questions of their safety for the fetus are unresolved. Calcium channel blockers may offer another modality of intravenous treatment, but their safety and efficacy are unproven.

Additional Therapeutic Considerations. Glucocorticoids administered to the mother between 27–33 weeks of gestation with intact membranes have been reported to reduce the incidence of neonatal respiratory distress. Protocols involve treatment regimens of betamethasone, 12 mg given intramuscularly twice 24 hours apart; dexamethasone, 5 mg given intramuscularly twice daily for four doses; or hydrocortisone, 500 mg given intramuscularly every 6 hours for a total of four doses. These doses are usually repeated every 7 days as long as preterm delivery seems likely. Use of glucocorticoids is an option that could be considered.

Specimens from patients who present with preterm premature rupture of membranes should be cultured for group B streptococci. If positive, patients should be treated intrapartum (see Chapter 5).

Intrapartum Care: Labor and Delivery

Childbirth is a unique family experience, and the obstetric staff should strive to make the patient and her support person comfortable and informed throughout the process. In large measure, the patient's and the family's perception of the intrapartum experience is determined by information provided during the antepartum period, particularly in regard to the normal physiologic processes occurring within both mother and fetus. The father or supporting person puts into practice the principles that were learned regarding the conduct of labor. Physical contact of the newborn with the parents in the delivery room may enhance future relationships, and hospital personnel should be encouraged, where feasible, to facilitate family interaction and to support the desire of the family to be together.

Because a significant proportion of patients may experience intrapartum complications, ongoing surveillance of the mother and fetus is essential. The hospital, including a birth center within the hospital complex, provides the safest setting for labor, delivery, and the postpartum period. The collection and analysis of data on the safety and outcome of deliveries in other settings, such as free-standing centers, have been problematic, as documented by a study conducted by the National Academy of Sciences. Until such data are available, the use of other settings is not encouraged. There may be exceptional situations, however, that require special programs, such as those in geographically isolated areas. Any facility providing obstetric care should have the services listed as essential components for a level I hospital (Chapter 1).

Admission

It is desirable for the initial history, physical findings, and laboratory data to be transmitted to the hospital soon after the first prenatal visit. Between 32–36 weeks of gestation, the patient's prenatal care record should be updated in the hospital's labor registration area. When the patient is admitted for labor and delivery, her prenatal care record should be reviewed; pertinent information from this record should be recorded on the admission note (eg, blood group and Rh type, presence of irregular antibodies or hepatitis B surface antigen, results of serologic and other diagnostic tests, and therapeutic measures prescribed). It is not necessary to repeat blood typing and screening tests at the time of hospital admission for labor and delivery if they were performed during the antepartum period and did not indicate the presence of antibodies, if the report is in the hospital records, and if there is no indication that the patient may need a blood transfusion. The nursing admission note should include the following information:

- Reason for admission
- Date and time of the patient's arrival and notification of the physician
- Time seen by the physician
- Condition of both mother and fetus
- Labor and membrane status

Patients in labor, with premature rupture of membranes, or with vaginal bleeding should be admitted directly to the labor and delivery suite. Occasionally, obstetric patients who are not in labor but who require special intensive care may also be admitted to this area. The admission of a patient in prodromal labor with no complications may be deferred, and she may be allowed to ambulate or wait in a more casual, comfortable area. Patients who have a transmissible infection, discharging skin lesions, diarrhea, or purulent vaginal discharge should be admitted to a specific labor, delivery, and recovery area where isolation techniques can be implemented according to established hospital policy (see also Chapter 6).

When a patient has had a recent examination and is not at high risk, the evaluation of her condition at admission may be restricted to an interval history and pertinent physical examination. Attention should be focused on the onset of contractions, status of membranes, bleeding, fetal activity, history of allergies, time and content of the most recent food ingestion, and the use of any medication.

The admitting physical examination should include determination of the patient's blood pressure, pulse, and temperature. The frequency, duration, and quality of the uterine contractions should be documented. The estimated fetal weight and fetal heart rate should be determined and documented on admission. Fetal well-being should be evaluated, and the method of assessment used should be determined by departmental policy.

When there are no complications or contraindications, as established by departmental protocol, qualified nursing personnel may perform the initial pelvic examination. Cervical dilatation, effacement, fetal presentation, and station should be documented. A urine sample should be tested to determine the presence of protein and glucose. The physician responsible for the patient's care should be informed of her status so that a decision can be made regarding present risk and further management. The timing of the physician's arrival in the labor area is determined by this information and by hospital policy. If anesthesia other than local or pudendal is likely to be needed or desired, anesthesia personnel should be informed soon after the patient's admission. After the results of the patient examination, as well as diagnostic and therapeutic orders, have been noted on the record, any necessary consent forms should be signed and attached to the record.

Departmental policies and physician preference concerning admission procedures such as taking of showers, placement of intravenous lines, use of electronic fetal heart rate monitoring, and ambulatory restrictions should take into consideration the patient's needs and desires. The use of drugs for analgesia and anesthesia during labor and delivery also should depend on the needs and desires of the patient and on the judgment of the attending physician.

Patients who have had no prenatal care should be considered to be at higher risk for special problems, especially infectious disease (such as syphilis, hepatitis B, and human immune deficiency virus [HIV]). A patient who has not had an orientation visit to the labor and delivery area as part of a childbirth education program or who is unfamiliar with monitoring techniques will require a careful explanation of what will happen during labor.

Analgesia and Anesthesia

Control of discomfort and pain during labor and delivery is a necessary part of good obstetric practice. Pain can be controlled by pharmacologic means or by techniques learned by the patient in a childbirth preparation program. The choice and availability of analgesic and anesthetic techniques depend on the experience and judgment of the anesthesiologist, the circumstances of labor and delivery, and the personal preferences of the obstetrician and the patient.

Of the various pharmacologic methods used for pain relief during labor and delivery, lumbar epidural block is the most effective and least depressant, allowing for an alert, participating mother. Continuous infusions of dilute solutions of local anesthetics (either alone or in combination with low doses of opioids) provide a more constant level of analgesia than intermittent injections of more concentrated solutions. They also may be associated with less motor blockade, a decreased risk of local anesthetic toxicity, and fewer acute hemodynamic changes. Lumbar epidural block may be complicated by maternal hypotension and has also been associated with an increased incidence of operative delivery. However, by using newer techniques in which less motor blockade is produced, this association may no longer be seen.

Parenteral opioids safely provide varying degrees of pain relief; however, high doses are potentially depressant to both mother and fetus. Similarly, a low concentration of inhalation analgesia may be useful in certain circumstances. Barbiturates, tranquilizers, and scopolamine have no analgesic qualities and are also potentially depressant. At the time of delivery, local infiltration and pudendal block are safe techniques; however, they do not provide total pain relief and, thus, are not sufficient for all vaginal births. Spinal anesthesia can provide adequate pain relief and muscle relaxation for nearly all vaginal births, but, unlike continuous lumbar epidural block, spinal anesthesia is useful only at the time of birth; other measures are required for pain control during the first stage of labor. Most important, general anesthesia is rarely necessary for vaginal births and should be used only for specific indications.

Paracervical block, when used for pain relief for labor, may result in fetal bradycardia. For this reason, close monitoring of the fetal heart rate is recommended when this method of pain relief is used. Because of adverse reactions, bupivacaine is contraindicated for use in paracervical block.

For uncomplicated cesarean deliveries, properly administered regional or general anesthesia is effective and has little adverse effect on the newborn. Because of the risks to the mother associated with intubation and the possibility of aspiration during the induction of general anesthesia, regional anesthesia may be the safer technique and should be available to all patients. The advantages and disadvantages of both techniques should be discussed with the patient as completely as possible.

If properly chosen and administered, analgesia or anesthesia during labor and delivery has little or no effect on the physiologic status of the neonate. At present, there is no evidence that the administration of analgesia or anesthesia during childbirth has a significant effect on the child's later mental and neurologic development.

Because the safety of obstetric anesthesia depends principally on the skill of the anesthesiologist, and because obstetric anesthesia must be considered emergency anesthesia, it demands a competence in personnel and an availability of equipment similar to or greater than that required for elective surgical procedures. Regional anesthesia in obstetrics should be initiated and maintained only by providers approved through the institutional credentialing process to administer or supervise the administration of obstetric anesthesia and must be qualified to manage anesthetic complications. An obstetrician who is appropriately trained to do so may administer the anesthesia if granted privileges for these procedures. It is preferable, however, for an anesthesiologist or anesthetist to provide this care so that the obstetrician can give undivided attention to the delivery. All obstetricians should be trained in the use of infiltration anesthesia. It is the responsibility of the director of anesthesia services to make recommendations regarding the clinical privileges of all anesthesia service personnel. If obstetric anesthesia is provided by obstetricians, the director of anesthesia services should participate with a representative of the obstetric department in the formulation of mechanisms designed to provide uniform quality of anesthesia services throughout the hospital. Specific recommendations regarding these mechanisms are provided in the Accreditation Manual for Hospitals. The directors of departments providing anesthesia services are responsible for implementing processes to monitor and evaluate the quality and appropriateness of these services in their respective departments.

Regional anesthesia should be administered only after the patient has been examined by a qualified individual, and the maternal and fetal status and progress of labor have been evaluated by a physician with credentials in obstetrics who concurs with the initiation of the anesthetic and is readily available to supervise the labor and manage any obstetric complications that may arise. When regional anesthesia is administered during labor, the patient's vital signs should be monitored at regular intervals by a qualified member of the health care team.

The following factors place a woman at anesthesia risk and should be communicated to the anesthesia care provider to permit formulation of a management plan in advance of the delivery:

- Marked obesity
- Severe facial and neck edema
- Extremely short stature
- Difficulty opening her mouth
- Small mandible or protuberant teeth, or both
- Arthritis of the neck
- Short neck
- Anatomic abnormalities of the face or mouth
- Large thyroid
- Asthma
- Severe preeclampsia
- Significant medical or obstetric complications, eg, eclampsia
- History of problems attributable to prior anesthetics

Because aspiration is a significant leading cause of anesthetic-related maternal mortality and morbidity, and because the aspiration of acidic gastric contents (pH less than 2.5) is more harmful than the aspiration of less acidic gastric contents, the prophylactic administration of an antacid before the induction of a major regional or general anesthesia is appropriate. Particulate antacids may be harmful if aspirated; therefore, a clear antacid, such as 0.3 mol/L sodium citrate or a similar preparation, may be a safer choice.

On rare occasions it may be impossible to intubate an obstetric patient following induction of general anesthesia. As emergency percutaneous transtracheal/cricothyroid ventilation may be lifesaving in this circumstance, the necessary equipment for performing this procedure should be immediately available whenever general anesthesia is administered.

Labor

Term

After the patient in labor has been admitted and her status initially evaluated, ongoing intrapartum surveillance is necessary; the level of surveillance may vary according to predetermined risk factors. A physician should see the patient within a reasonable period of time, as determined by her obstetric and other medical conditions, after her admission to the hospital. Each hospital should develop maximal allowable physician response times for high-risk and low-risk patients. The patient may be permitted to ambulate with the knowledge and consent of the attending physician. General care during labor should provide optimal patient comfort in addition to optimal fetal and maternal safety.

For each shift in the labor and delivery area, the patient should be introduced to the nurse responsible for her care. A designated member of the obstetric team should be responsible for observing the patient, following the progress of labor, and recording the patient's vital signs and fetal heart rate on the labor record. The physician who is responsible for the patient's care should be kept informed of her progress and notified immediately of any abnormality. He or she should be readily available when the patient is in the active phase of labor.

For the patient without identifiable risks, assessment of the quality of uterine contractions, in conjunction with vaginal examinations, should be adequate to monitor the progress of labor and to detect abnormalities. The patient's temperature and pulse should be recorded every 4 hours, more often if indicated. Maternal blood pressure should be taken and recorded regularly. The patient should be encouraged to void at least every 3 hours during labor. The amount of fluid intake should be recorded. Any new significant symptom or sign (eg, excessive vaginal bleeding or pain, or meconium-stained amniotic fluid) should be evaluated by the responsible provider.

Patients should not ingest anything by mouth during labor except for small sips of water, ice chips, or preparations to moisten the mouth and lips. Hydration and nourishment during a long labor should be provided by means of the intravenous administration of fluids; this measure also minimizes acidemia and electrolyte imbalance.

Vaginal examinations should be kept to a minimum and conducted with careful attention to the use of a clean technique. This is particularly important if the membranes are ruptured. The use of a sterile lubricant may reduce discomfort from the examination. Sterile, water-soluble lubricants are recommended for vaginal examinations during pregnancy. Because lubricants containing antiseptics such as povidone-iodine or hexachlorophene have not been shown to decrease the frequency of infections, and because the antiseptic compounds may be absorbed through the vaginal mucosa and may be harmful to the fetus, they are not appropriate agents for vaginal antisepsis.

The intensity and method of fetal heart rate monitoring used during labor should be based on risk factors and delineated by departmental policy. It has been shown that with a 1:1 nurse/patient ratio, intermittent auscultation at intervals of 15 minutes during the active phase of the first stage of labor and 5 minutes during the second stage is equivalent to continuous electronic fetal heart rate monitoring. Thus, when risk factors are present during labor or when intensified monitoring is elected, the fetal heart rate should be assessed by one of these methods according to the following guidelines:

- During the active phase of the first stage of labor, the fetal heart rate should be evaluated and recorded at least every 15 minutes, preferably following a uterine contraction, when intermittent auscultation is used. If continuous electronic fetal heart rate monitoring is used, with or without external or internal uterine contraction monitoring, the tracing should be evaluated at least every 15 minutes.

- During the second stage of labor, the fetal heart rate should be evaluated and recorded at least every 5 minutes when auscultation is used and should be evaluated at least every 5 minutes when electronic fetal heart rate monitoring is used.

There are no data to demonstrate optimal time intervals for intermittent auscultation for low-risk patients. The standard practice is to evaluate and record the fetal heart rate at least every 30 minutes following a contraction in the active phase of the first stage of labor and at least every 15 minutes in the second stage of labor.

When electronic fetal heart rate monitoring is selected as the method of fetal assessment, the physician and obstetric personnel attending the patient should be qualified to identify and interpret abnormalities. It is appropriate for physicians and nurses to use the descriptive terms that have been given to fetal monitoring patterns (eg, accelerations and early, late, or variable decelerations) in chart documentation and verbal communication. Consultation with professionals should be sought when the staff responsible for patient care needs assistance in interpreting fetal heart characteristics. In the event of differences of interpretation among professionals involved in the care of specific patients, an established hospital policy for the resolution of such a conflict should be followed.

Internal uterine pressure monitoring can provide important information regarding the strength and frequency of contractions. This technique may help to record uterine activity more accurately when indicated, but it is not required for all patients in labor.

Notation of such items as physician or nurse presence, the patient's position in the bed, cervical status, oxygen or drug administration, hypertension or hypotension, fever, amniotomy, color of the amniotic fluid, and Valsalva efforts provides a detailed and graphic documentation of the course of events during labor. Abnormal findings should be identified and appropriate intervention implemented. It is especially important that when a change in fetal heart rate patterns has been noted, a subsequent return to normal patterns be documented as well. Each tracing should include the patient's name, hospital number, date and time of admission and delivery, EDD, gravida/para, and other data required for medical records. All tracings should be stored in a way that makes them readily retrievable.

Preterm

When patients are admitted in preterm labor, they should be assessed for gestational age and the possibility of fetal or maternal infection should be determined. Particular attention should be given to the care of mothers and infants when delivery will occur at the early limits of viability. Protocols should be developed for the use of tocolytic agents, including the indications for their use and the management of their side effects.

In the presence of premature rupture of membranes and an immature fetus without signs of infection, it is reasonable to observe the patient rather than to induce labor. Management of preterm labor in the presence of premature rupture of membranes remains controversial. The risk of chorioamnionitis and fetal infection must often be weighed against the risks associated with the delivery of a premature infant. If amniotic fluid has pooled in the vagina, it can be examined for evidence of fetal lung maturity (phosphatidyl glycerol determination). Speculum examination can permit visualization of the cervix and culturing for group B streptococci (see Chapter 5). A digital examination should be avoided if the patient is not in labor.

Decisions concerning route and location of delivery should be based on the neonate's chances of survival and risk of morbidity. Such statistics need to be individualized for the patient population, capability of the center, and concurrent risk factors; thus, the decisions governing clinical care cannot be standardized but vary according to provider, location, and patient population. Tertiary care centers should make this information available for their referral area.

All preterm deliveries occurring after 24 weeks of gestation should occur in a setting capable of neonatal resuscitation, with an individual qualified to perform resuscitation present. It is difficult to predict gestational age with sufficient accuracy around 24 weeks, when a week or less in error can mean a major difference in the chances of survival. Appropriate pediatric consultation should be considered in these circumstances. Local and regional statistics for neonatal survival at a given gestational age (by best obstetric estimate) should help guide obstetric decisions about place and mode of delivery and intensity of fetal monitoring. The mother's risk of morbidity and mortality must also be weighed against the chances of intact neonatal survival.

The pediatric service should be notified of the possibility of a preterm delivery; if necessary, transfer to a hospital with facilities for the care of these mothers and infants should be arranged. Survival rates of preterm infants born in a facility with an intensive care nursery are higher than those of birth-weight-controlled infants born in a smaller facility and transported into a tertiary care center. Thus, if time is available to effect safe maternal transport, any woman likely to deliver an infant too small or too sick to be well cared for in her intended hospital may be considered for transport to a facility better able to care for the infant. It is usually best if obstetrician and pediatrician can agree in advance on the approximate gestational age at which deliveries can safely take place in their hospital. The value of maternal transport should be balanced against the risks. Transports should not interfere with prompt initiation of therapy. For example, maternal hypertension, significant bleeding, fetal distress, or advanced labor may contraindicate maternal transport. Delivery in a relatively small medical facility is much safer than birth of a preterm infant or maternal deterioration in a car, ambulance, or helicopter at some distance from any obstetric or pediatric care.

Induction and Augmentation

Labor may be induced or augmented with oxytocin only after a thorough examination of both mother and fetus and indications for and methods of induction or augmentation have been documented.

A physician who has privileges to perform cesarean deliveries should be readily available to respond should problems arise. This should be documented in the record. A physician or qualified nurse should examine the patient vaginally prior to the initiation of oxytocin infusion. Personnel who are familiar with the effects of oxytocin and able to identify both maternal and fetal complications should be in attendance during the administration of oxytocin.

Each hospital's department of obstetrics and gynecology should determine the indications for induction and augmentation of labor, and should establish a written protocol for the preparation and administration of the oxytocin solution. This protocol should delineate methods for maternal and fetal assessment. Monitoring the fetal heart rate should be similar to that recommended for high-risk patients in active labor (see description of term labor above). Oxytocin should be administered only intravenously, with a device that permits precise control of the flow rate.

Delivery

Specific preparation for delivery should be instituted at a time dictated by the patient's parity, labor progress, fetal presentation, labor complications, and anesthesia management. At least one member of the nursing staff should be present in the delivery room throughout the delivery. Under no circumstances should any attempt be made to delay the birth by physical restraint or anesthesia.

Episiotomy is used to protect the perineum; it is not always necessary, however, and should not be considered routine. The presence of a short perineum, a large baby, and the need to shorten the second stage of labor are some of the current indications for its use.

Whichever method of monitoring (auscultation or continuous electronic fetal monitoring) is being used in patients who will undergo cesarean delivery, it should be continued until the abdominal preparation is begun. If internal monitoring is being used, the scalp electrode should remain attached to the fetus and the monitoring equipment until the abdominal preparation is complete.

Cesarean Delivery

Any hospital that provides labor and delivery services should be equipped to perform an emergency cesarean delivery. The nursing, anesthesia, neonatal resuscitation, and obstetric personnel required must be either in the hospital or readily available. It should be possible, when indicated, to begin the operation within 30 minutes of the time that the decision is made to operate. Not all indications for a cesarean delivery will require a 30-minute response time. Examples of those mandating the need for expeditious delivery may include hemorrhage from placenta previa, abruptio placentae, prolapsed umbilical cord, and uterine rupture.

Surgical packs, solutions, and other materials and supplies should be kept sealed but conveniently arranged so that the instrument table can be ready almost immediately for an obstetric emergency.

Elective repeat cesarean delivery does not necessarily constitute a high-risk situation for the neonate. Because the duties of the surgical and anesthesia team may preclude their caring for a neonate, another qualified person skilled in neonatal resuscitation should be present in the delivery room to care for the neonate. The qualifications needed should be defined by the hospital's medical staff. Prior to an elective repeat cesarean delivery, fetal maturity should be established in accordance with the criteria previously stated.

Vaginal Birth After Cesarean Delivery

Recent data show that 50–80% of patients with a low transverse uterine incision from one previous cesarean birth who attempt to deliver vaginally have successful vaginal births. Data also show that maternal and perinatal mortality rates associated with vaginal delivery after cesarean delivery are no higher than those for repeat cesarean delivery. Although uterine rupture can occur, it is rarely catastrophic because of the availability of modern fetal monitoring, anesthesia, and obstetric support services. A successful vaginal delivery not only eliminates operative and postoperative complications, but also shortens the patient's hospital stay.

Unless there are contraindications to vaginal delivery, women who have had one previous low transverse cesarean delivery should be counseled and encouraged to attempt labor in their current pregnancy. A woman who has had two or more previous cesarean deliveries with low transverse incisions and who wishes to attempt vaginal birth should not be discouraged from doing so in the absence of contraindications. A woman should not be forced to undergo a trial of labor. Certain social, geographic, and past obstetric complications may justify the patient's electing to have a repeat cesarean birth.

Operative Vaginal Delivery

Forceps and vacuum extraction are safe and valuable tools in the management of labor. The definitions and indications for vacuum are consistent with those for forceps:

- *Station:* The relationship of the estimated distances, in centimeters, between the leading bony portion of the fetal head and the level of the maternal ischial spines. In classifying forceps procedures, the level of engagement of the fetal head must be stated as precisely as possible. Engagement of the head occurs when the biparietal diameter has passed through the pelvic inlet and is clinically diagnosed when the leading bony portion of the fetal head is at or below the level of the ischial spines (station 0 or more).

- *Outlet forceps:* The application of forceps when 1) the scalp is visible at the introitus without separating the labia, 2) the fetal skull has reached the pelvic floor, 3) the sagittal suture is in the anterior–posterior diameter or in the right or left occiput anterior or posterior position, and 4) the fetal head is at or on the perineum. According to this definition, rotation cannot exceed 45°. There is no difference in perinatal outcome when deliveries involving the use of outlet forceps are compared with similar spontaneous deliveries, and there are no data to support the concept that rotating the head on the pelvic floor 45° or less increases morbidity. Forceps delivery under these conditions may be desirable to shorten the second stage of labor.

- *Low forceps:* The application of forceps when the leading point of the skull is at station +2 or more. Low forceps has two subdivisions: 1) rotation 45° or less (eg, left or right occipitoanterior to occiput anterior, left or right occipitoposterior to occiput posterior) and 2) rotation more than 45°.

- *Midforceps:* The application of forceps when the head is engaged but the leading point of the skull is above station +2. Under very unusual circumstances, such as the sudden onset of severe fetal or maternal compromise, application of forceps above station +2 may be attempted while simultaneously initiating preparations for a cesarean delivery in the event that the forceps maneuver is unsuccessful. Under no circumstances, however, should forceps be applied to an unengaged presenting part or when the cervix is not completely dilated.

The indications for the forceps operation, including the position and station of the vertex at the time of application of the forceps, should be specified in a detailed operative description in the patient's medical record. These indications include the following:

- Shortening the second stage of labor: Outlet forceps may be used to shorten the second stage of labor in the best interests of the mother or the fetus, as long as the criteria for outlet forceps are met.

- Prolonged second stage: The following durations are approximate; when these intervals are exceeded, the risks and benefits of allowing labor to continue should be assessed and documented:

  — Nulliparous: More than 3 hours with a regional anesthetic or more than 2 hours without a regional anesthetic

— Parous: More than 2 hours with a regional anesthetic or more than 1 hour without a regional anesthetic
- Fetal stress
- Maternal indications (eg, cardiac, exhaustion)

The following conditions are required for forceps operations:

- An experienced person performing or supervising the procedure
- Assessment of maternal–fetal size relationship
- Adequate anesthesia
- Willingness to abandon attempt if forceps procedure does not proceed easily

Care of the Neonate

The first minutes of life may determine the quality of that life. The need for prompt, organized, and skilled response to immediate neonatal emergencies requires written policies delineating responsibility for immediate newborn care, resuscitation, selection and maintenance of necessary equipment, and training of personnel in proper techniques.

Routine Care

The delivering physician or nurse–midwife is responsible for providing immediate postdelivery care of the newborn and for ascertaining that the newborn adaptations to extrauterine life are proceeding normally unless the care has been transferred. The hospital rules and regulations should include protocols for the transfer of medical care of the neonate in both routine and emergency circumstances. Routine care of the healthy newborn may be delegated to appropriately trained nurses, or transferred to a family physician or pediatrician.

Information to be transmitted to the physician caring for the infant after delivery includes both the infant's and the mother's name and medical record number; the mother's blood type, serology result, rubella status, hepatitis B screen result, diabetes screen, exposure to group B streptococci, and record of substance abuse; and the presence of fetal anomalies.

At least one person skilled in initiating resuscitation should be present at every delivery. The skills and responsibilities of that individual should be defined at the institutional level.

Resuscitation

Recognition and immediate resuscitation of a distressed neonate requires an organized plan of action and the immediate availability of qualified personnel and equipment as described in the American Academy of Pediatrics and the American Heart Association *Textbook of Neonatal Resuscitation*. Responsibility for identification and resuscitation of a distressed neonate should be assigned to a qualified individual, who may be a physician or an appropriately trained nurse–midwife, labor and delivery nurse, nurse–anesthetist, nursery nurse, or respiratory therapist. The provision of services and equipment for resuscitation should be planned jointly by the directors of the departments of obstetrics, anesthesia, and pediatrics, with the approval of the medical staff. A physician should be designated to assume primary responsibility for initiating, supervising, and reviewing the plan for management of depressed neonates in the delivery room. The following factors should be considered in this plan:

- A list of maternal and fetal complications that require the presence in the delivery room of someone specifically qualified in all aspects of newborn resuscitation should be developed.
- Individuals qualified to perform neonatal resuscitation should demonstrate the following capabilities:
  — Skills in rapid and accurate evaluation of the newborn condition, including Apgar scoring.
  — Knowledge of the pathogenesis and causes of a low Apgar score (eg, hypoxia, drugs, hypovolemia, trauma, anomalies, infections, and prematurity), as well as specific indications for resuscitation.
  — Skills in airway management (eg, laryngoscopy, endotracheal intubation, suctioning of the airway), artificial ventilation, cardiac massage, emergency administration of drugs and fluids, and maintenance of thermal stability. The ability to recognize and decompress tension pneumothorax by needle aspiration is also a desirable skill.
- Procedures should be developed to ensure the readiness of equipment and personnel and to provide for intermittent review and evaluation of the effectiveness of the system.
- Contingency plans should be established for multiple births and other unusual circumstances.
- A physician for the neonate need not be present at a delivery provided that no complications are anticipated and another skilled individual is present to care for the neonate.

- The resuscitation steps should be documented in the records.

Apgar Score

Apgar scores (Table 3-3) should be obtained at 1 minute and 5 minutes after the complete birth of the neonate. If the 5-minute score is less than 7, it is useful to obtain additional scores every 5 minutes until 20 minutes have passed or until two successive scores of 7 or greater are obtained.

When necessary, resuscitation should be initiated before the 1-minute Apgar score is obtained. The Apgar score should be assigned by someone not directly involved in resuscitating the neonate. Low scores (less than 3), especially those associated with a delay in the return of tone, are useful in identifying the neonate who is significantly depressed; the change between the 1-minute score and the 5-minute score is useful in assessing the efficacy of resuscitation. Low Apgar scores, however, should be used neither as the sole factor in defining neonatal asphyxia nor as a single predictor of later mortality or developmental disability. Other parameters such as abnormal fetal status, umbilical cord or scalp blood pH, signs of organ injury, and occurrence and nature of seizures are useful additional data for determination of neonatal status at birth and for predicting outcomes.

If a low Apgar score is anticipated or assigned, rapid assessment of the neonate's condition is necessary in order to delineate a plan of care. Umbilical cord blood gas and pH analyses may help to distinguish metabolic acidemia secondary to hypoxia from other causes of low Apgar scores in the depressed neonate.

Maintenance of Body Temperature

Immediately following delivery, the neonate should be put in a warm place and dried completely. Drying the neonate with prewarmed towels

Table 3-3. Apgar Score

Sign	0	1	2
Heart rate	Absent	Slow (<100 beats/min)	100 beats/min
Respirations	Absent	Weak cry; hypoventilation	Good, strong cry
Muscle tone	Limp	Some flexion	Active motion
Reflex irritability (response to brisk slap on soles of feet)	No response	Grimace	Cough or sneeze
Color	Blue or pale	Body pink; extremities blue	Completely pink

immediately after birth reduces evaporative heat loss. It is recommended that a radiant warmer with a servocontrol mechanism be placed in the resuscitation area, because such devices allow easy access to the neonate during resuscitation procedures.

Suctioning

The neonate's mouth may be suctioned gently to remove excess mucus or blood. Although clear mucus is suctioned from the mouth routinely in most centers, there is no evidence to support the value of this practice. Vigorous suctioning of the posterior pharynx should be avoided, as this may produce significant bradycardia.

If there is meconium in the amniotic fluid, the mouth and hypopharynx should be thoroughly suctioned with a mechanical device before delivery of the shoulders in a cephalic presentation and immediately after delivery of the head in a breech presentation. In the presence of thick or particulate meconium, the larynx should be visualized and any meconium present removed. If meconium is present and the infant is depressed, the clinician should intubate the trachea and suction to remove meconium or other aspirated material from beneath the glottis. If the infant is vigorous, the indication for vocal cord visualization and tracheal aspiration of meconium is less clear. It has been suggested that for the vigorous and spontaneously breathing infant who may have aspirated the meconium, less indication exists for aggressive removal. Furthermore, injury to the vocal cords is more likely to occur in attempting to intubate a vigorous infant. When using a mechanical suction apparatus, the suction pressure should be set so that when the suction tubing is occluded the negative pressure does not exceed 100 mm Hg.

Ventilation

The normal neonate breathes within seconds of delivery and has established regular respiration within 1 minute of delivery. A flaccid neonate who is not breathing spontaneously and whose heart rate is less than 80 beats per minute requires immediate positive pressure ventilation. A bag and mask can often provide effective ventilation (Fig. 3-1), but it may be difficult to use this method in premature neonates with noncompliant lungs. If the neonate's heart rate does not rise promptly to more than 60–80 beats per minute, endotracheal intubation is required.

Before applying positive pressure ventilation, it is important to ensure that the airway has been cleared. The head should be placed in a sniffing

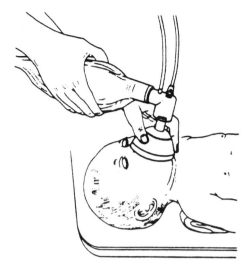

Fig. 3-1. Assisted ventilation of the newborn with bag and mask. Reproduced with permission. Textbook of Neonatal Resuscitation, 1987. © American Heart Association

position, with care to avoid hyperextension of the neck. The middle or fourth finger should be placed behind the posterior ramus of the mandible, thrusting the mandible forward; no fingers (or any part of the mask) should rest on the soft tissues of the neck. Initial lung inflation may require 30–40 cm H_2O, and 15–20 cm H_2O is often adequate for succeeding breaths, which should be provided at a rate of 40 per minute. With rare exceptions, depressed neonates respond promptly to adequate ventilation, and this is the only resuscitation maneuver required.

Symmetric movement of the apices of the chest; equal breath sounds (heard in the axillae); and improvement in heart rate, color, and muscle tone indicate satisfactory ventilation. The response of the heart rate is the most useful and readily measurable criterion of adequate resuscitation. If the response to ventilation is not prompt, the seal between the face and the mask or the position of the endotracheal tube should be checked. If chest movement and breath sounds appear satisfactory in an intubated neonate, yet the neonate is not responding, the position of the endotracheal tube should be checked by direct visualization of the larynx with a laryngoscope.

External Cardiac Massage

If the heart rate does not rise promptly to more than 60–80 beats per minute after effective ventilation with oxygen, external cardiac massage should be instituted while ventilation is continued. Two techniques are illustrated

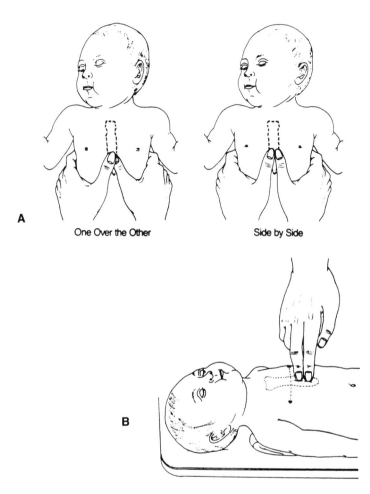

A

One Over the Other   Side by Side

B

Fig. 3-2. Techniques for external cardiac massage. A. The chest is encircled with both hands and the thumbs compress the sternum. B. The tips of the middle finger and either the index or ring finger of one hand are used for compression. Reproduced with permission. Textbook of Neonatal Resuscitation, 1987. © American Heart Association

in Figure 3-2. Chest compressions should be carried out at a rate of 120 beats per minute to a depth of ½–¾ inch. If there is no response in the heart rate, appropriate drug therapy (and volume expansion, if indicated) should be instituted.

Drugs and Volume Expansion

The use of drugs for resuscitation of the neonate is rarely necessary in the delivery room. When drugs are needed, they should not be administered until ventilation and circulation have been established. The emergency route of administration is the umbilical vein. The infusion of epinephrine into the trachea via an endotracheal tube may also be an effective route of administration.

Acidosis. Severely depressed neonates may have a combined metabolic and respiratory acidosis. The treatment of acidosis is treatment of the cause. Thus, respiratory acidosis, which is the result of hypoventilation, is treated by providing positive pressure ventilation. Metabolic acidosis is the result of hypoxemia or hypoperfusion, and the correction of these factors should correct the acidosis.

Significant acidemia is detrimental to myocardial function in the hypoxic heart. Sodium bicarbonate may be useful in a prolonged resuscitation to help correct a documented metabolic acidosis, but its use is discouraged in brief arrests or episodes of bradycardia. In the absence of adequate ventilation, sodium bicarbonate will not improve blood pH significantly. One molar sodium (8.4%) bicarbonate should not be used. One-half molar sodium (4.2%) bicarbonate or lesser concentrations are acceptable.

Bradycardia. Epinephrine hydrochloride may be indicated for bradycardia that persists after adequate ventilation and cardiac massage.

Hypovolemia. It is important to recognize that most severely depressed neonates are not hypovolemic and that there may be potential hazards (eg, intracranial hemorrhage) to rapid volume expansion. Conditions associated with hypovolemia include significant hemorrhage from the fetoplacental unit (eg, vasa praevia, fetomaternal bleeding) and compression of the umbilical cord.

If significant hypovolemia is suspected, it should be treated with repeated infusions of volume expanders (10 ml/kg). The neonate's response should be assessed after each infusion. Therapy is stopped when tissue perfusion is adequate.

Narcotic-Induced Respiratory Depression. If respiratory depression is the result of narcotics administered to the mother prior to delivery, naloxone hydrochloride, 0.1 mg/kg, may be administered to the neonate in conjunction with assisted ventilation.

Resources and Recommended Reading

American Academy of Pediatrics. Committee on Drugs. Naloxone dosage and route of administration for infants and children: addendum to emergency drug doses for infants and children. Pediatrics 1990; 86(3):484–485

American Academy of Pediatrics, Committee on Fetus and Newborn. Use and abuse of the Apgar score. Pediatrics 1986;78(6):1148–1149

American College of Obstetricians and Gynecologists. Alpha-Fetoprotein. ACOG Technical Bulletin 154. Washington, DC: ACOG, 1991

American College of Obstetricians and Gynecologists. Antenatal diagnosis of genetic disorders. ACOG Technical Bulletin 108. Washington, DC: ACOG, 1987

American College of Obstetricians and Gynecologists. Intrapartum fetal heart rate monitoring. ACOG Technical Bulletin 132. Washington, DC: ACOG, 1989

American College of Obstetricians and Gynecologists. Preterm labor. ACOG Technical Bulletin 133. Washington DC: ACOG, 1989

American College of Obstetricians and Gynecologists. Ultrasound imaging in pregnancy. ACOG Committee Opinion 96. Washington, DC: ACOG, 1991

American Society of Anesthesiologists. Guidelines for conduction anesthesia in obstetrics. Park Ridge, IL: ASA, 1990

American Society of Anesthesiologists. Standards for basic intra-operative monitoring. Park Ridge, IL: ASA, 1989

American Society of Anesthesiologists. Standards for postanesthesia care. Park Ridge, IL: ASA, 1988

Bloom RS, Cropley C, eds. The textbook of neonatal resuscitation. Dallas: American Heart Association, 1987

Briggs GG, Freeman RK, Yaffe SJ. Drugs in pregnancy and lactation. 3rd ed. Baltimore: Williams & Wilkins, 1990

Joint Commission on Accreditation of Health Care Organizations. Accreditation Manual for Hospitals, 1991. Oak Brook Terrace, IL: JCAHCO, 1990

Knight GJ, Palomaki GE, Haddow JE. Use of maternal serum alpha-fetoprotein measurements to screen for Down's syndrome. Clin Obstet Gynecol 1988;31(2):306–327

Lenke RR, Levy HL. Maternal phenylketonuria: results of dietary therapy. Am J Obstet Gynecol 1982;142(5):548–553

Main DM, Gabbe SG, Richardson D, Strong S. Can preterm deliveries be prevented? Am J Obstet Gynecol 1985;151(7): 892–898

Rhoads GG, Jackson LG, Schlesselman SE, de la Cruz FF, Desnik RJ, Golbus MS, et al. The safety and efficacy of chorionic villus sampling for early prenatal diagnosis of cytogenetic abnormalities. N Engl J Med 1989;320(10):609–617

Tucker JM, Goldenberg RL, Davis RO, Copper RL, Winkler CL, Hauth JC. Etiologies of preterm birth in an indigent population: is prevention a logical expectation? Obstet Gynecol 1991;77(3):343–347

CHAPTER 4

POSTPARTUM AND FOLLOW-UP CARE

Postpartum hospitalization has several purposes: to identify maternal and neonatal complications, to provide professional assistance during the time when the mother is most likely to be uncomfortable, and to allow adequate time for instruction so that the parents may return home with reasonable competence and confidence. The continuum of perinatal care that began in the antepartum period should be reinforced during hospitalization to ensure that care extends beyond discharge. A multidisciplinary, collaborative approach is frequently used to promote this continuity, as well as to ensure that care is comprehensive.

The Postpartum Period

Immediate Care

Postpartum care begins immediately after delivery, in the recovery area or birthing room where the woman can be observed for postpartum complications, such as hemorrhage or hematoma formation. Stabilization of the neonate usually occurs within the first 12 hours after birth, during which time the condition of the neonate is closely monitored. Neonates who appear to be healthy need not leave their mother for this stabilization period if the facilities needed for their observation are in the mother's recovery or postpartum area and there is adequate nursing personnel to observe and document the status of the neonate. The father or other supporting person may remain with the new mother during the immediate postpartum period. Parents should be encouraged to interact with the neonate unless such interaction is precluded by maternal or neonatal complications.

Maternal Considerations

During the period of observation immediately after delivery, matenal blood pressure and pulse should be taken and recorded every 15 minutes for the first hour, more frequently if the patient's condition warrants. The amount of vaginal bleeding should be evaluated often and the uterine fundus palpated often to check for size to determine whether it is well contracted. The administration of a dilute solution of oxytocin by intravenous drip after delivery of the placenta reduces the incidence of postpartum hemorrhage. For postpartum hemorrhage due to uterine atony not responsive to oxytocin or ergot alkaloids, 15α-methyl-prostaglandin $F_{2\alpha}$ should be available. If vaginal bleeding occurs or if the patient complains of perineal pain, the cause of the bleeding or pain should be determined by careful palpation of the uterus and by inspection and palpation of the perineum, vagina, and cervix for lacerations or hematoma formation.

Following major regional or general anesthesia for either vaginal or cesarean delivery, the patient should be observed in an appropriately staffed and equipped postanesthesia care unit or equivalent area, or an appropriately equipped labor/delivery/recovery room, until she has recovered from the anesthetic. Following cesarean delivery, the same standards for postanesthesia care should apply to patients receiving major obstetric anesthesia as are applied to other surgical patients receiving major anesthesia. Staff assigned to the recovery area should have no other obligation. There should be a policy to ensure the availability in the facility of a physician capable of managing anesthetic complications and providing cardiopulmonary resuscitation for patients in the postanesthesia care unit. The patient should be discharged from the recovery area only at the discretion of the attending physician or the anesthesiologist in charge. A record of vital signs should be maintained and additional signs or events monitored and recorded as they occur.

If a woman has had a major anesthetic for her delivery and the anesthetic can be continued safely, there is no contraindication to proceeding with a tubal sterilization in the immediate postpartum period if the mother's condition is satisfactory and no maternal complication suggests that deferral is necessary. If tubal sterilization necessitates the induction of anesthesia (regional or general), the anesthesiologist should carefully evaluate the patient's condition. If there is any indication of a neonatal problem, the timing of this elective procedure should be reevaluated. The decision as to when to proceed with anesthesia and surgery should be based on the anesthesiologist's assessment of the patient and judgment of the relative risks and benefits for that patient.

Neonatal Considerations

Following an initial evaluation of the neonate's condition, a care plan should be established and the neonate carefully observed for the next 6–12 hours. Feeding can be initiated as soon as possible after delivery.

During the stabilization period, temperature, heart and respiratory rates, skin color, adequacy of peripheral circulation, type of respiration, level of consciousness, tone, and activity should be monitored and recorded at least once every 30 minutes until the neonate's condition has remained stable for 2 hours. Following these observations, the neonate who has no identified problem may be placed in the newborn nursery or in the mother's room for continued surveillance and care until discharge. If the neonate remains with the mother, the physician or nurse should assess and document the neonate's condition according to the routine of the transitional nursery. Any conditions that require special attention, such as respiratory distress or hypothermia, should be noted and actions taken to correct a problem should be documented in the baby's record. After appropriate initial care in the resuscitation area, neonates who at birth are sick, small, or at high risk of becoming sick (as determined by history or physical examination) should be transferred to an intermediate or intensive care area.

Identification. While the newborn is still in the delivery room, two identical bands that indicate the mother's admission number, the neonate's sex, and the date and time of birth or information specified in hospital policy should be placed on the wrist or ankle. The nurse in the delivery room should be responsible for preparing and securely fastening these identification bands on the neonate. Footprinting and fingerprinting are not adequate methods of patient identification.

The birth records and identification bands should be checked before the neonate leaves the delivery room. When the neonate is taken to the nursery, both the delivery room nurse and the admitting nurse should check the identification bands and birth records, verify the sex of the neonate, and sign the neonate's record. The admitting nurse should fill out the bassinet card and attach it to the bassinet. Later, when the neonate is shown to the mother, she should be asked to verify the information on the identification bands and the sex of the neonate. It is imperative that delivery room and nursery personnel be meticulous in the preparation and placement of the neonate's identification bands.

Risk Assessment. As soon as possible, no later than 2 hours after birth, admitting personnel should evaluate the neonate's status and assess risks. Necessary clinical data that were unavailable initially should be either obtained or requested at this time. Risks can be assessed through the history and physical examination as documented on the antepartum and intrapartum records. These records should accompany the neonatal record.

The neonate's physician should examine the apparently normal neonate no later than 12–18 hours after birth and within 24 hours before discharge from the hospital. The results of these examinations should be recorded on the neonate's chart and discussed with the parents.

Birth Weight/Gestational Age Classification. The neonate's gestational age should be calculated from the mother's menstrual history, physical examination, obstetric milestones noted during pregnancy, and the obstetrician's assessment of gestational age (Fig. 4-1). Currently, the most reliable way to confirm the estimated date of delivery is by ultrasound examination at less than 20 weeks of gestation. Any marked discrepancy between the presumed duration of pregnancy and the physical and neurologic findings in the neonate should be evident on the chart.

Data from each neonate should be plotted on a birth weight–gestational age chart that indicates whether the neonate is small, average, or large for gestational age. The determination of gestational age and its relationship to weight can be used in the identification of neonates at risk for illness. For example, neonates who are either large or small for their gestational age are at relatively increased risk for hypoglycemia and polycythemia, and appropriate tests (eg, serum glucose screen or hematocrit determination) are indicated.

Cord Blood. The Rh group of the cord blood should be determined and Coombs antibody tested routinely at the time of delivery if the mother is Rho(D) negative. If the mother was not recently tested, blood typing, Rh determination, and serologic tests for syphilis should be done on cord blood or on blood drawn from the neonate before discharge. Requirements for testing may differ with the population of patients served.

Eye Care. The application of two drops of 1% silver nitrate in single-dose containers or a 1–2-cm ribbon of sterile ophthalmic ointment containing tetracycline (1%) or erythromycin (0.5%) in single-use tubes is acceptable prophylaxis against gonococcal ophthalmia neonatorum. Care should be taken to ensure that the agent reaches all parts of the conjunctival sac. The eyes should not be irrigated with saline or distilled water after instillation of any of these agents; however, after 1 minute, excess solution or ointment can be wiped away with sterile cotton. Instillation may be delayed up to 1 hour following birth. Infants born by cesarean delivery also should receive eye prophylaxis. The effectiveness of erythromycin or tetracycline in the prevention of opthalmia caused by penicillinase-producing *Neisseria gonorrhoeae* is not established. For gonococcal isolates known to be penicillin sensitive, intramuscular penicillin G (50,000 U for full-term

	0	1	2	3	4	5
Neuromuscular maturity						
Posture						
Square window (wrist)	90°	60°	45°	30°	0°	
Arm recoil	180°		100°-180°	90°-100°	<90°	
Popliteal angle	180°	160°	130°	110°	90°	<90°
Scarf sign						
Heel to ear						
Physical maturity						
Skin	gelatinous red, transparent	smooth pink, visible veins	superficial peeling &/or rash, few veins	cracking pale area, rare veins	parchment, deep cracking, no vessels	leathery, cracked, wrinkled
Lanugo	none	abundant	thinning	bald areas	mostly bald	
Plantar creases	no crease	faint red marks	anterior transverse crease only	creases ant. 2/3	creases cover entire sole	
Breast	barely percept.	flat areola, no bud	stippled areola, 1-2 mm bud	raised areola, 3-4 mm bud	full areola, 5-10 mm bud	
Ear	pinna flat, stays folded	sl. curved pinna, soft with slow recoil	well-curv. pinna, soft but ready recoil	formed & firm with instant recoil	thick cartilage, ear stiff	
Genitals ♂	scrotum empty no rugae		testes descending, few rugae	testes down, good rugae	testes pendulous, deep rugae	
Genitals ♀	prominent clitoris & labia minora		majora & minora equally prominent	majora large, minora small	clitoris & minora completely covered	

Apgar_____1 min_____5 min
Age at exam _____ (hr)
Race _____ Sex _____
B.D. _____
LMP _____
EDC _____
Gestational age
  by dates _____(wk)
Gestational age
  by exam_____(wk)
Birth weight _____(g)
    _____ percentile
Length_____(cm)
    _____percentile
Head circum._____(cm)
    _____ percentile
Clin. dist.____None____Mild
    _____ Mod.____ Severe

Maturity rating

Score	Weeks
5	26
10	28
15	30
20	32
25	34
30	36
35	38
40	40
45	42
50	44

Fig. 4-1. Assessment of neonatal maturity. The assessment is quickly and easily performed because the chart includes measures of physical maturity and measures of passive tone but not active tone. Items are arranged so that a neonate who scored 2 on each item would be assessed as being at 34 weeks of gestation. Physical maturity is most accurately assessed in the minutes or hour or so following birth. The score for each item is indicated at the top of the vertical column. However, neuromuscular maturity may be misleading in the depressed neonate. Thus, neuromuscular maturity rating should be repeated after a day or two. The sum of scores on all the items of physical and neuromuscular maturity provides a maturity in weeks (see lower right). The physical maturity score times two provides an approximation of maturity rating in weeks. Ballard JL, Kazmaier K, Driver M. A simplified assessment of gestational age. Pediatr Res 1977;2(4):374

infants and 20,000 U for low-birth-weight infants) also is effective for prophylaxis. No topical regimen has proven efficacy in the prevention of chlamydial conjunctivitis.

Vitamin K. To prevent vitamin K-dependent hemorrhagic disease and coagulation disorders, every neonate should receive a single parenteral dose of 0.5–1 mg of natural vitamin K_1 oxide (phytonadione) within 1 hour of birth. Although studies generally show that oral administration of vitamin K to the mother has some efficacy, parenteral administration to the neonate is preferred.

Subsequent Care

Specific postpartum policies and procedures should be established through cooperative efforts of the medical and nursing staff. While in the postpartum unit, the mother should be taught how to care for herself and her neonate, and problems related to her general health should be discussed. Healthy neonates born after uncomplicated pregnancies should be assigned to a care plan that includes appropriate observation for the stabilization period and the remainder of the hospital stay. Neonates with identified problems or risk factors usually require individualized care plans.

The physician should note postpartum orders on the patient's chart. Routine postpartum orders may be used, but they should be printed or written on the chart, reviewed and modified as necessary for the particular patient, and signed by the physician before the patient's transfer to the postpartum unit. When a birthing, labor/delivery/recovery, or labor/delivery/recovery/postpartum room is used, the same standards of care should apply as in the traditional setting.

Maternal Considerations

When the patient is taken to her postpartum room, her vital signs, the status of the uterine fundus, and the rate of bleeding should be reassessed and recorded. This assessment should be repeated at regular intervals for the next several hours.

Bed Rest, Ambulation, and Diet. Bed rest is recommended for only a brief time, just long enough to allow the new mother to sleep, regain her strength, and recover from the effects of the analgesic or anesthetic agents that she may have received during labor. It may be necessary to administer intravenous fluids for hydration. Because early ambulation has been shown to decrease the incidence of subsequent thrombophlebitis, the patient should be encouraged to walk, with assistance, as soon as she feels able. The patient should not attempt to get out of bed initially without the help of an attendant. The mother may have a full diet as soon as she desires it, unless her physician gives other orders. The mother may shower after she is able to walk.

Care of the Vulva. The patient should be taught to cleanse the vulva from anterior vulva to perineum and anus rather than in the reverse direction. The application of an ice bag may help to reduce edema and pain during the first 24 hours after repair of episiotomy. Orally administered analgesics are often required and are usually sufficient for relief of discomfort from episiotomy. Pain that is not relieved by such medication suggests hematoma formation and mandates a careful examination of the vulva, vagina, and rectum. Beginning 24 hours after delivery, moist heat in the form of a warm sitz bath can be applied to reduce local discomfort and promote healing.

Care of the Bladder. Women often have difficulty voiding immediately after delivery, possibly because of trauma to the bladder during labor and delivery, regional anesthesia, or pain from the episiotomy site. In addition, the diuresis that sometimes follows delivery may distend the bladder before the patient is aware of it. To ensure adequate emptying of the bladder, the patient should be checked frequently during the first 24 hours after delivery, with particular attention to displacement of the uterine fundus and any indication of a fluid-filled bladder above the symphysis. Every effort should be made to help the patient void spontaneously; however, single catheterization may be necessary. If the patient continues to find voiding difficult, the use of an indwelling catheter may be preferable to repeated catheterization.

Care of the Breasts. The mother's decision about breast-feeding her newborn determines the appropriate care of the breasts. Breast care for a woman who chooses to breast-feed is outlined in Chapter 7. The woman who does not desire to breast-feed should be reassured that stopping the milk production is not a major problem. During the stage of engorgement, the breasts become painful and should be supported with a well-fitting brassiere. Ice packs or small doses of analgesics may be required to relieve discomfort during this 12–24-hour period.

Temperature Elevation. The condition of all postpartum patients with an elevated temperature should be evaluated and appropriate cultures taken (see Chapter 6). The nursery should be notified if the mother develops a fever, especially within the first 24 hours, so that the neonate can be examined for potential infection. In most cases there is no need for the neonate to be separated from the mother.

Postpartum Analgesia. Following vaginal delivery, analgesia may be necessary to relieve episiotomy pain and facilitate maternal mobility. Most mothers experience considerable pain in the first 24 hours following cesarean birth. Although in the past intramuscular injections of narcotics have been used most frequently in this circumstance, newer techniques such as spinal or epidural opiates and patient-controlled analgesia may provide better pain relief and greater patient satisfaction. Regardless of their route of administration, opioids can potentially cause respiratory depression; thus adequate supervision and monitoring should be ensured for all patients receiving these drugs on the postpartum ward.

Immunization: Rh Immune Globulin (RhIg) and Rubella. An unsensitized Rho(D)-negative woman who delivers an Rho(D)- or Du-positive neonate should receive 300 μg of RhIg postpartum, ideally within 72 hours, even when RhIg has been administered in the antepartum period. This dose may be inadequate in circumstances where there is potential fetal–maternal hemorrhage, such as abruptio placentae, placenta previa, intrauterine manipulation (as may be required for the delivery of twins), manual removal of the placenta, cesarean delivery, precipitous delivery, multifetal gestation, and hydramnios. In these cases, laboratory analysis should be performed to detect excessive maternal–fetal hemorrhage and thus determine the proper dosage. If indicated, additional RhIg should be administered. If a patient is determined to be Du positive prior to pregnancy, she does not need RhIg.

A patient who has been identified as rubella susceptible should receive the rubella vaccine in the postpartum period. Rubella vaccine can be administered after delivery prior to discharge, even if the patient is breast-feeding.

Neonatal Considerations

The condition of the neonate should be evaluated on admission to the nursery. This evaluation should include a review of the neonate's identification, the mother's health prior to pregnancy and during the prenatal and intrapartum periods, the neonate's condition at birth, and the neonate's success in adapting to extrauterine life. Based on this initial assessment, an individualized care plan should be established. Observations should be made and recorded every 8 hours until discharge; the specific times of observation should be recorded as well.

It is advisable to develop nursery guidelines to delineate those conditions (eg, low birth weight, small size for gestational age, or questionable clinical status) that require specific actions by nurses or immediate notification of the physician. Clinical conditions such as maternal drug abuse, maternal fever or infection, or low Apgar scores are associated with increased risk for neonatal illness and should prompt immediate notification of the physician. The obstetrician should be advised of the baby's status, particularly if problems arise.

Observation. The neonate should be observed for any signs of illness:

- Temperature instability
- Change in activity, including refusal of feedings
- Unusual skin color
- Abnormal cardiac or respiratory rate and rhythm
- Delayed or abnormal stooling or voiding

The normal full-term neonate passes meconium within the first 24 hours of life. If the full-term neonate has not passed meconium by 48 hours of age, the lower gastrointestinal tract may be obstructed. Urine is normally passed within the first 12 hours. Failure to void in the first 24 hours may indicate genitourinary obstruction or abnormality or dehydration.

Nursery Environment. Concerns have been expressed that neonates, especially those that are premature or chronically ill, may be adversely affected by modern nursery environments. Many nurseries are constantly illuminated at high foot-candle levels and have noise levels that are many decibels higher than desirable. While physicians and nursing personnel stay in the nursery environment for intervals of hours at most, some neonates remain there for weeks or even months.

Pending development of more specific information, prudence suggests that attempts be made to control excessive stimulation and to correct the lack of variation in nursery environments. High-intensity noise should be avoided. (Regulations of the Occupational Safety and Health Administration [OSHA] do not permit a level of more than 80 dB for longer than 8 hours for an adult.) Light intensity of 60 ft-c is adequate for observation, whereas 100 ft-c of light is required for the performance of most procedures; additional lighting can be provided when necessary. Activities of personnel and stimulation of babies for feeding or procedures can be altered to allow for diurnal cycles and rest or nap intervals.

Weighing. Each neonate should be weighed at least daily. The neonate must be kept warm during weighing. The scale pan should be covered with a clean paper before each neonate is weighed. The accuracy of the nursery scales should be checked once a month.

Clothing. Most neonates require only a cotton shirt or gown without buttons in addition to a soft diaper. They may be clothed only in a diaper during hot weather if the nursery is not air-conditioned. A supply of soft, clean, cotton clothing, bed pads, sheets, and blankets should be kept at the bedside. Nontoxic dyes should be used to mark clothing, blankets, or other items used in the care of newborns.

Bathing. Skin care, including bathing, may be important for the health and appearance of the individual neonate and for infection control within the nursery. The first bath should be postponed until thermal stability is assured. The medical and nursing services of each hospital should develop guidelines regarding the time of the first bath, circumstances and method of skin cleansing, and role of personnel and parents. Supervised involvement of new parents, including discussion of bathing in health education classes, is recommended. The use of special equipment, such as radiant warmers, is recommended for premature and unstable infants.

Neonatal Screening. All neonates should be entered into an adequate screening program that includes, as a minimum, tests for the persistent hyperphenylalaninemias (PHP), including phenylketonuria (PKU), and for congenital hypothyroidism in its various forms. In addition, many states screen for hemoglobinopathies, including sickle cell disease.

A screening program should include the following components:

- Participation of all neonates
- Notification of parents
- Reliable and prompt performance of the screening test
- Prompt follow-up of subjects whose tests have positive results
- Accurate diagnosis of subjects with confirmed positive test results
- Appropriate counseling and treatment of patients

The program should conform with the following recommendations:

- A blood sample should be obtained from every neonate prior to discharge or transfer. Neonates whose siblings have PHP/PKU or congenital hypothyroidism merit special priority in the collection of blood samples. For PHP/PKU, an adequate sample from a full-term neonate is defined as heel blood obtained as close as possible to the time of discharge from the nursery (cord blood is not sufficient); for congenital hypothyroidism, it is cord blood at birth or heel blood at discharge. For neonates who are premature, being fed parenterally, or being treated for illness, a blood sample obtained at or near 7 days of age is adequate.

- Neonates initially screened before 24 hours of age should be rescreened for PHP/PKU because cases may be missed by a screening test so soon after delivery. The repeat screening test should be completed no later than the third week of life.

- Screening methods should be standardized to promote accurate analysis. The level considered abnormal should be defined. The specificity of the test should be monitored regularly, which requires a high volume of samples per unit of time. The analytic component in the program should be centralized to enhance ongoing evaluation of efficiency, accuracy, participation, and adequacy.

- All patients with PHP should be investigated to rule out the tetrahydrobiopterin-deficient forms of PKU.

- Systematic follow-up of neonates with positive results on screening tests for congenital hypothyroidism is necessary to evaluate the efficacy of efforts to ameliorate the effects of this condition and to manage premature infants with transiently low thyroxine values.

The incidence of polycythemia and hyperviscosity is estimated to be approximately 3% of the newborn population. The condition occurs most commonly among high-risk infants such as those with diabetic mothers, intrauterine growth retardation, perinatal asphyxia, and twin-to-twin transfusion recipients. Screening for polycythemia and hyperviscosity should be considered in these high-risk infants; in low-risk infants screening for this condition may be at the discretion of the institution. The appropriate timing of screening for this condition is during the first 6–12 hours of life. Capillary blood samples may be used. It should be noted that, in newborns, the capillary hematocrit is generally higher than the venous hematocrit.

Hypoglycemia. Neonatal hypoglycemia, a common metabolic disorder, may result in significant neurologic sequelae, especially in the symptomatic infant, if left untreated. Therefore, the rationale for glucose screening in the newborn infant is to identify and treat this metabolic condition as early as possible.

The indications and criteria for neonatal glucose screening are less well defined. In certain groups of high-risk infants who have a higher incidence of hypoglycemia than the normal population, neonatal glucose screening is highly recommended. These groups include infants of diabetic mothers; infants with intrauterine growth retardation, perinatal hypoxia, polycythemia, severe erythroblastosis fetalis, or a family history of hypoglycemia; and infants who have clinical signs and symptoms suggestive of hypoglycemia, such as irritability, lethargy, periodic cyanosis and apnea, poor feeding, unexplained respiratory distress, and abnormal cry.

The timing of the glucose screening is variable depending on the clinical condition. For instance, in infants of diabetic mothers, the nadir of blood glucose concentration occurs sometime during the first 2 hours of life. Thus, it is appropriate to initiate the screening for hypoglycemia during this period. On the other hand, the onset of hypoglycemia in infants with polycythemia may occur later in the first day.

Methods for glucose screening in infants also are not well established. Glucose analysis using a laboratory-quality glucose analyzer at the bedside has proven reliable and accurate. However, at the present time it is impractical to expect every nursery to have this method available on the unit. Glucose oxidase reagent strips are more commonly used for screening. These are screening devices, and the values obtained from them should never be used as a basis for the diagnosis of neonatal hypoglycemia. If hypoglycemia is diagnosed by a reagent strip method in an asymptomatic infant, the low blood glucose concentration should be confirmed by a laboratory glucose oxidase method before treatment is initiated. In the symptomatic infant, treatment can be initiated with glucose infusion for confirmation of hypoglycemia provided that a blood sample was obtained prior to infusion.

It is highly recommended that each institution establish a written policy for the indications, timing, methods, and procedures for the screening of hypoglycemia in newborn infants.

Inborn Errors of Metabolism. Although screening reveals many inborn errors of metabolism, screening is inadequate for many metabolic diseases because severe signs and symptoms develop before screening results are available. Symptomatic inborn errors of metabolism of the neonate are rare, but when considered as a group, they represent an important cause of morbidity among full-term infants who had no antepartum or intrapartum risk factors. Inborn errors of metabolism appear in premature and full-term infants with an approximately equal frequency; therefore, more than 90% of symptomatic inborn errors of metabolism in the neonatal period are found in full-term infants. Because effective therapy is available for many of these diseases, early diagnosis and treatment may mitigate or prevent permanent neurologic sequelae. Physicians should become familiar with their state requirements for screening.

Circumcision. Newborn circumcision is an elective procedure to be performed only in healthy and stable infants. The exact incidence of postcircumcision complication is not known, but the data to date indicate that the rate is low and that the most common complications are local infection and bleeding. Circumcision may also result in a reduced incidence of urinary tract infection, although prospectively collected data in this regard are lacking. Circumcision may be done under local anesthesia. However, local anesthesia does add an element of risk; thus, it would be prudent to obtain more data from a large, controlled trial before recommending routine use of local anesthesia during newborn circumcision.

Visiting

The father or supporting person may be with the mother as much as desired throughout the intrapartum and postpartum periods within the constraints of acceptable standards of care. Whenever possible, parents of ,ieonates in the continuing care, intermediate care, or intensive care areas should be allowed unrestricted visits. Provisions should be made for feeding (particularly breast-feeding), handling, and holding these neonates. Visiting policies for fathers should be formulated to be as flexible and liberal as possible and followed consistently.

Sibling visits may be appropriate in the early labor and postpartum periods based on local policy. Contact with the mother and newborn in the hospital helps prepare the siblings for the new family member and is reassuring for younger children. Physical contact of siblings with neonates is a topic of current concern because of the possible transmission of viral infectious diseases. If siblings are allowed to have direct contact with the newborn, the visit may take place in the mother's private room or in a special sibling visitation area if the mother is not in a private room. Thorough hand-washing should be required. Parents should share the responsibility of preventing the exposure of their newborn to a sibling with a contagious illness. Contact of the newborn with children other than siblings should be avoided.

No adverse effects of sibling visitation in neonatal intensive care units have been noted, but more study is needed before a general recommendation can be made. An institution that allows sibling visitation to the neonatal intensive care unit should have clearly defined written policies and procedures based on information presently available. The following guidelines may serve as the basis for policy formulation:

- Siblings should not have been exposed to known communicable diseases (eg, chickenpox).
- Siblings should not have fever or symptoms of acute illness, such as upper respiratory infection or gastroenteritis.
- Children should be prepared in advance for their visit.
- Parents are responsible for ensuring that children are properly supervised by an adult throughout their hospital visit.
- Thorough hand-washing should be required.

Because available data are limited, there is a need for continued evaluation and reporting of the risks and benefits of sibling visitation. This should include both psychologic and infectious disease factors. Institutions that have not introduced sibling visitation should consider the opportunity to use controlled trials to study the effects of these programs.

Education and Psychosocial Factors

The reduction in the average length of a patient's hospital stay to 2–3 days or even less has compromised the opportunity for parent education. Hospital resources that have traditionally been extended to parents can no longer be accommodated within the shortened hospital stay. Physicians should be willing to accept, understand, and respond to parent inquiries that arise throughout the perinatal period and make every effort to ensure that educational aspects of care are provided prior to and following hospitalization.

Closed-circuit television films previewed and approved by the obstetric and pediatric staff, printed materials, and counseling by hospital personnel (eg, postpartum and nursery nurses, registered dietitians/nutritionists, and physical therapists) have been helpful to parents. Other beneficial activities are group or individual educational sessions held regularly during the postpartum period to teach and discuss patient self-care, including exercises and self-examination of the breasts; parent–infant relationships; infant care, including bathing and feeding; and child growth and development. Family planning techniques appropriate to the patient's needs and desires should be explained in detail.

The newborn undergoes rapid changes in physiology that should be explained to the parents. The neonate's cardiovascular, pulmonary, renal, and neurologic maturation should be observed by the parents with the guidance of qualified personnel. Parents should be familiar with normal and abnormal changes in wake–sleep patterns, temperature, respiration, voiding, stooling, and the appearance of the skin. They should also observe and become familiar with the behavior, temperament, and neurologic capabilities of the newborn. Some believe that parents should also learn infant cardiopulmonary resuscitation techniques.

During the postpartum hospital stay, health care personnel can provide the mother with professional assistance when she is most likely to be uncomfortable and can help her to anticipate how she may feel once she is home. The new mother may be unsure of the normal physical changes that occur after delivery and of her ability to care for the newborn. The mother should be evaluated when she is with her infant(s) to identify problems she is having so that appropriate instructions with education can be provided prior to discharge. Prenatal instructions given to prepare the family for the infant's care at home should also be reinforced.

Both in-hospital and community agencies may assist the family. Information on public and private groups that give assistance and circumstances under which these organizations may be asked for assistance should be available in the hospital. Various sources may include the following:

- The in-hospital social service department should be an integral part of the interdisciplinary effort to coordinate hospital and discharge activities, to obtain public or private assistance, and to render psychosocial support.

- Members of the Visiting Nurses Association may be available to visit the home to assess the parents' child-rearing skills, the home environment, maternal emotional stability, and infant status and development. Under the physician's direction, these nurses may administer drugs or provide other types of therapy.

- Certain groups may be available to lend support and provide education on special activities (eg, breast-feeding).

Discharge

Prior to discharge a discussion should be held between the physician or another health care provider and the mother (and father, if possible) about any expected perinatal problems and ways to cope with them. Plans for future and immediate care, as well as instructions to follow in the event of an emergency or complication, should be discussed.

Maternal Considerations

Prior to discharge, the patient should be informed of normal postpartum events, including the changes in the lochial pattern that she should expect in the first few weeks; the range of activities that she may reasonably undertake; the care of the breasts, perineum, and bladder; dietary needs, particularly if she is breast-feeding; the recommended amount of exercise; emotional responses; and observations that she should report to the physician (eg, temperature elevation, chills, leg pains, or increased vaginal bleeding). The length of convalescence based on the type of delivery should be discussed, and patients should be counseled to avoid abdominal straining. Patients who have abnormal bleeding or signs of infection or fever should not be discharged. It is helpful to reinforce oral discussion with written information.

Methods of contraception should be fully reviewed and implemented. A diaphragm cannot be fitted adequately during the immediate postpartum period. If there are no contraindications, however, oral contraceptive use may begin right after delivery. Breast-feeding mothers may start using oral contraceptives once their milk flow is established. Patients for whom the use of oral contraceptives is contraindicated or patients who prefer other methods of contraception, such as foam and condoms, should be instructed in the use of these other methods.

The time at which coitus may be resumed after delivery is controversial. If resumed too soon, coitus may cause vaginal laceration and pain. Risks of hemorrhage and infection are minimal after approximately 2 weeks postpartum; by this time, the uterus has involuted markedly, and the endometrium and cervix have begun to reepithelialize. Thereafter, coitus may be resumed based on the patient's desire and comfort, and after contraceptive issues have been resolved. Sexual difficulties are common in the early months after childbirth. Scarring at the episiotomy site may cause the woman some discomfort during intercourse for 1–3 months. In the lactating woman, the vagina is often atrophic, and lubrication during sexual excitement may be unsatisfactory. Furthermore, the demands of infant care alter the couple's ability to find the time previously allocated to physical intimacy.

At the time of discharge, arrangements should be made for postpartum follow-up examination, and specific instructions should be conveyed to the mother. The following points should be reviewed with the mother or, preferably, with both parents:

- Condition of the neonate
- Immediate needs of the neonate (eg, feeding methods and environmental supports)
- Roles of the obstetrician, pediatrician, and other members of the health care team concerned with the continuous medical care of the mother and neonate
- Availability of support systems, including psychosocial support
- Instructions to follow in the event of a complication or emergency
- Feeding techniques; skin care, including cord care; temperature assessment and measurement with the thermometer; and assessment of neonatal well-being and recognition of illness
- Reasonable expectations for the future
- Importance of maintaining immunization begun with initial dose of hepatitis B vaccine

When no complications are present, the postpartum hospital stay ranges from 48 hours for vaginal delivery to 96 hours for cesarean birth, excluding the day of delivery. When the mother is discharged early, especially within 24 hours of delivery, certain criteria should be met:

- The mother should have had an uncomplicated vaginal delivery following a normal antepartum course and should have been observed after delivery for a sufficient time to ensure that her condition is stable. Pertinent laboratory data, including a postpartum determination of hemoglobin or hematocrit level and, if not previously obtained, ABO blood group and Rh typing, should have been obtained. If indicated, the appropriate amount of RhIg should have been administered.
- Family members or other support person(s) should be available to the mother for the first few days following discharge.
- The mother should be aware of possible complications and should have been instructed to notify the appropriate practitioner, as necessary.
- Procedures for readmission of obstetric patients should be consistent with hospital policy, as well as local and state regulations.

The medical and nursing staff need to be sensitive to potential problems associated with early discharge and to develop mechanisms to address patient questions that arise after discharge.

Early Infant Discharge and Follow-up

The nursery stay is planned to allow the identification of early problems and to reinforce instructions in preparation for the infant's care at home. Complications often are not predictable by prenatal and intrapartum events. Because many neonatal problems do not become apparent until several days after birth, there is an element of medical risk in early neonatal discharge. Although most problems are manifest during the first 6 hours, data suggest that readmissions may be more common when early (by 48 hours) or very early (by 24 hours) discharge programs are instituted. With these observations in mind, the following criteria for early infant discharge are recommended:

- The course of antepartum, intrapartum, and postpartum care, for both mother and fetus, should be without complications.
- Maternal readiness to assume independent responsibility for her newborn should be assured by demonstration of skills and abilities such as feeding techniques, skin and cord care, measurement of temperature with a thermometer, and ability to assess infant well-being and recognize common neonatal illnesses. Family members who will care for the child should attend prenatal childbirth education or infant care classes, in which problems of the first days after birth are discussed.
- The infant should be delivered at term, be of appropriate birth weight, and found normal by examination.
- The infant should be able to maintain thermal homeostasis as well as suck and swallow normally.
- A physician-directed source of continuing medical care for both mother and baby should be identified and arrangements made for the baby to be examined within 48 hours of discharge.
- Laboratory data should be reviewed to include:
  —Maternal testing for syphilis and hepatitis B surface antigen
  —Cord or infant blood type and direct Coombs test (if the mother is Rho(D) negative, or is type O, or if screening has not been performed for maternal antibodies)

—Hemoglobin or hematocrit and blood glucose determinations as clinically indicated

—Screening tests required by law

- Initial hepatitis B vaccine should be administered.

At the initial follow-up visit, within 48 hours of discharge, the following assessments of the infant should be made:

- Evaluation of condition by history and physical examination to include evidences of adequate nutrition and hydration, normal stool pattern, degree of jaundice, quality of mother–infant interaction, and details of infant behavior
- Review of laboratory data obtained before discharge
- Screening tests for PKU, hypothyroidism, and other metabolic disorders, as indicated by state law and clinical judgment
- Planning for health maintenance, to include arrangements for emergency services, preventive care and immunizations, periodic evaluations, and necessary screening

High-Risk Infants

Each hospital should develop guidelines for the discharge of high-risk infants that may include the following criteria:

- The infant should be physiologically stable and should be able to maintain body temperature without cold stress when the amount of clothing worn and the room temperature are appropriate.
- The infant should be able to tolerate oral feeding by breast or bottle. If the infant's clinical condition precludes normal nipple feeding, the parents or other care providers should be instructed in an alternative feeding program.
- The infant should be gaining weight steadily at the time of discharge.
- The infant should be free of apnea prior to discharge or be receiving appropriate treatment.
- The physician or discharge planner should have confirmed parental competence (eg, ability to administer medications).
- The home situation should be considered appropriate.

It is essential to have a well-coordinated plan for the discharge and follow-up care of high-risk infants:

- A complete physical examination should be performed prior to discharge in order to identify problems that require specialized monitoring (eg, heart murmur, apnea, seizures, atypical head growth pattern) and to provide data on which to base future assessments.

- Immunization against diphtheria, tetanus, and pertussis (DTP) can be initiated in medically and neurologically stable preterm infants who have attained a chronologic age of 2 months. The status of this immunization should be assessed before discharge. Although the response of premature infants to *Haemophilus influenzae* type B vaccine is currently unknown, the first immunization should be given at 2 months of chronologic age.

- All preterm infants should be screened for anemia prior to discharge. It may be necessary to provide supplemental vitamins, iron, or blood transfusions.

- Infants with history of deafness in the family, rubella exposure in the first trimester, maxillofacial anomalies, birth weight less than 1,000 g, meningitis, or hyperbilirubinemia treated with exchange transfusion may require referral for audiometric evaluation.

- Low-birth-weight infants (ie, those who were delivered at less than 35 weeks of gestation or weighed less than 1,800 g at birth) who receive oxygen supplementation are at an increased risk for retinopathy of prematurity and should undergo an ophthalmologic evaluation prior to discharge or at 5–7 weeks of age if still hospitalized. Infants who were born at less than 30 weeks of gestation or who weighed less than 1,300 g should also be examined regardless of oxygen exposure. The examination should be repeated according to the schedule appropriate to the original findings. Follow-up is recommended for those with significant active disease.

- Parents of infants with bronchopulmonary dysplasia require specific instruction in administering medications (eg, diuretics, bronchodilators) and feeding (eg, schedules, amount, technique, problem solving, and caloric supplements). They must be adequately trained to recognize signs of acute deterioration (eg, wheezing, congestion, distress) and to carry out cardiopulmonary resuscitation. Infants who continue to be oxygen dependent may be discharged if appropriate family and community resources are available and the infant is feeding adequately, growing, and able to maintain adequate oxygenation activity while receiving oxygen via nasal cannula at a rate no more than 1 L/min. Initial follow-up contact every 1–2 weeks is indicated.

- Informed consent should be obtained from their parents before infants are discharged with home apnea monitors. Parents of these infants require anticipatory guidance, training in infant cardio-pulmonary resuscitation, complete verbal and written explanation of the monitor, guidelines for home monitoring, and referral for follow-up services.

Legislation in most states mandates that infants and children from birth to age 4 years be restrained in appropriate car seats while in motor vehicles. A recent study has indicated, however, that infants with a current weight of less than 2,000 g are at an increased risk of oxygen desaturation and bradycardia when placed in a standard car seat. Parents should be alerted to this risk and should be counseled regarding alternatives, as described in the article by the American Academy of Pediatrics Committee on Injury and Poison Prevention, "Safe Transportation of Premature Infants."

Part of the discharge plan should include an assessment of the family's strengths and weaknesses. Appropriate referrals to any of the following ancillary services can then be initiated accordingly:

- Visiting nurse
- Social service
- Women, Infants, and Children (WIC) Program
- Mental health service
- Teen support services
- Parent support groups
- Early intervention services
- Respite care services

Follow-up Care

The physical and psychosocial status of the mother and neonate should be subject to ongoing assessment after discharge. The new mother needs personalized care during the postpartum period to hasten the development of a healthy mother–infant relationship and a sense of maternal confidence. Support and reassurance should be provided as the mother masters infant care tasks and adapts to her maternal role. Involving the father and encouraging him to participate in the neonate's care not only can provide additional support to the mother but also can enhance the father–infant relationship.

The postpartum period is a time of developmental adjustment for the whole family. Family members now have new roles and relationships, and an effort should be made to assess the progress of the family's adaptation. If a family member—mother, father, or sibling—finds it difficult to assume the new role, the health care team should arrange for sensitive, supportive assistance. This is particularly important for the teenaged mother, for whom it may be necessary to mobilize multiple resources within the community.

Maternal Considerations

Approximately 4–6 weeks after delivery, the woman should see her physician for postpartum review and examination. This interval may be modified according to the needs of the patient with medical, obstetric, or intercurrent complications.

Review at the first postpartum visit should include an interval history and physical examination to evaluate the patient's current status, as well as her adaptation to the newborn. Specific inquiries regarding breast-feeding should be made. The examination should include an evaluation of weight, blood pressure, breasts, and abdomen, as well as a pelvic examination. Methods of birth control should be reviewed.

Many women experience some degree of emotional lability in the weeks postpartum. If this persists or develops into true depression, intervention may be needed. The emotional status of women whose pregnancies had an abnormal outcome should also be reviewed. Counseling should address specific issues regarding their future health and pregnancies. For example, it may be necessary to discuss vaginal birth after a cesarean birth or the implications of diabetes, growth retardation, prematurity, hypertension, anomalies, or other conditions in which there is a risk of recurrence. Laboratory data should be obtained as indicated. This is a good time to review immunizations, including that against rubella, for those who are susceptible and did not receive the vaccine immediately postpartum, and to discuss any special problems. The patient should be encouraged to return for subsequent periodic examinations.

Neonatal Considerations

The frequency of follow-up visits for normal neonates varies with patient, locale, and community practices. Such visits are usually monthly in the first 3 months, bimonthly for the remainder of the first year, and three times during the second year. It is important that follow-up visits be regular and that good records of development be maintained.

The intervals of follow-up visits required by high-risk neonates should be determined by the needs of the individual infant and family. It may be necessary to examine some of these infants weekly or bimonthly at first. Neurologic, developmental, behavioral, and sensory status should be assessed more than once during the first year in high-risk infants to ensure early identification of problems and referral for remediation.

Physicians and others who provide follow-up care to mothers and infants should be aware of the physical, social, and psychologic factors associated with child abuse and its increasing occurrence. The following factors have been associated with child abuse:

- Prematurity
- Illness with long periods of hospitalization, especially in neonatal intensive care units
- Single parenthood
- Adolescent motherhood
- Closely spaced pregnancies
- Infrequent family visits to hospitalized infants

Children with a history of prematurity have been shown to have a greater incidence of irritability, hyperkinesis, and increased dependency. Prolonged hospitalization inevitably disrupts family relationships, particularly the parent–child relationship. Infants and parents with such a history require closer follow-up than does the average family. The interaction of the parents, especially the mother, with the infant should be evaluated periodically. The infant or child who fails to thrive may be a victim of neglect, if not outright abuse, and a causal relationship between neglect and failure to thrive should always be suspected. In every state those who provide health care to children are legally obligated to report suspected child abuse.

Assessments

Growth parameters should be assessed, with continued monitoring of the adequacy of weight gain, linear growth, and head growth. Growth should be plotted on standardized growth curves. Review of nutritional intake and calculation of caloric intake are helpful in case management.

The physical examination should include assessment of cardiac, pulmonary, and gastrointestinal status, as well as any hernias, anomalies, or orthopedic deformities. Parents of infants who were cared for in the neonatal intensive care unit are often concerned about minor scars secondary to procedures performed in the unit, and they benefit from reassurance.

Medication dosage should be reevaluated, dosages increased with weight gain and age, and blood levels monitored. Immunization status should be reviewed.

Families must be encouraged to obtain recommended follow-up vision and audiometric assessments when indicated. Audiometric assessment should include behavioral testing in a soundproof testing room and brain stem auditory-evoked-potential testing if behavioral results are inconclusive or if the infant is at risk for hearing loss. After the infant has reached 6 months of age, further assessment of receptive/expressive language skills, behavioral audiometry, and impedance testing are appropriate. Brain stem auditory-evoked-potential testing should be repeated if the results of these tests are equivocal.

In the primary physician's office, neurologic assessment should include an appraisal of muscle tone, reflexes, and visual and auditory responses. In addition, a standard developmental screening tool, such as the Denver Developmental Screening Test, should be used. When neurologic findings are suspicious or when developmental delays are suggested by screening, infants should be referred for more in-depth assessment, either to a neonatal follow-up program or to equivalent facilities or programs capable of providing detailed neurodevelopmental assessments.

In children 1–5 years of age whose conditions during the perinatal period (eg, severe depression, hypoglycemia, intracranial hemorrhage) increased the risk of neurologic defects, the following factors should be considered:

- Fine and gross motor abnormalities
- Visual–perceptual–motor abnormalities
- Receptive/expressive language delay
- Mild conductive or sensorineural hearing loss
- Hyperkinesis, attention deficit, behavior problems

Early Intervention

Infant stimulation and enrichment programs are designed to provide developmentally appropriate activities for children from birth to 3 years who are at risk for a variety of conditions that may interfere with their ability to lead a full and productive life. Infants who may be considered for such a program include those with motor handicaps, visual or auditory handicaps, orthopedic anomalies, syndromes associated with developmental delay, or known developmental delay. Intervention programs offer therapeutic guidelines for families, parent support groups, respite care programs, and innovative therapy modalities. Although there are no definitive data to confirm the beneficial effects of infant stimulation programs, there are indications that early intervention may improve the social adaptation of high-risk infants and their families.

Technology-Dependent Infants

In recent years, with improvements of survival rate among low-birth-weight infants, there has been an increasing number of infants who require cardiopulmonary monitoring for a considerable period of time at home. These children include those who suffer from bronchopulmonary dysplasia and those with persistent apnea. Many of the children with bronchopulmonary dysplasia may go home on oxygen and therefore require equipment to deliver oxygen at home, cardiopulmonary monitoring, and assessment of oxygen status by pulse oximeter. The appropriate management of these infants will require the coordinated team efforts of the tertiary care physicians, primary care physicians, discharge planning personnel, social workers, visiting nurses, and providers of home care products. It is desirable that the tertiary care personnel take responsibility for the coordinated plan for the management and follow-up of these children.

Resources and Recommended Reading

American Academy of Pediatrics, Ad Hoc Task Force on Care of Chronically Ill Infants and Children. Guidelines for home care of infants, children, and adolescents with chronic disease. Pediatrics 1984;74(3):434–436

American Academy of Pediatrics, Committee on Accident and Poison Prevention. Safe transportation of newborns discharged from the hospital. Pediatrics 1990;86(3):486–487

American Academy of Pediatrics, Committee on Fetus and Newborn. Postpartum (neonatal) sibling visitation. Pediatrics 1985;76(4):650

American Academy of Pediatrics, Committee on Genetics. Newborn screening fact sheets. Pediatrics 1989;83:449–464

American Academy of Pediatrics, Committee on Genetics. New issues in newborn screening for phenylketonuria and congenital hypothyroidism. Pediatrics 1982;69(1):104–106

American Academy of Pediatrics, Committee on Genetics. Prenatal diagnosis for pediatricians. Pediatrics 1989;84:741–744

American Academy of Pediatrics, Committee on Injury and Poison Prevention and Committee on Fetus and Newborn. Safe transportation of premature infants. Pediatrics 1991;871(1)120–122

American Academy of Pediatrics, Joint Committee on Infant Hearing. Position statement 1982. Pediatrics 1982;70(3):496–497

American Academy of Pediatrics. Report of the Task Force on Circumcision. Pediatrics 1989;84:388-391. See errata in Pediatrics 1989;85(5):761

American Academy of Pediatrics and American Thyroid Association. Newborn screening for congenital hypothyroidism: recommended guidelines. Pediatrics 1987;80(5):745–749

Caravella SJ, Clark DA, Dweck HS. Health codes for newborn care. Pediatrics 1987;80(1):1–5

Conrad PD, Sparks JW, Osberg I, Abrams L, Hay WW Jr. Clinical application of a new glucose analyzer in the neonatal intensive care unit: comparison with other methods. J Pediatr 1989;114:281–287

Cornblath M, Schwartz R, Aynsley-Green A, Lloyd JK. Hypoglycemia in infancy: the need for a rational definition. Pediatrics 1990;85:834–837

Freeman JM (ed). Prenatal and perinatal factors associated with brain disorders. National Institute of Child Health and Human Development and National Institute of Neurological and Communicative Disorders and Stroke. Washington, DC: US Government Printing Office, 1985 ; NIH Publication no. 85-1149

Hurt H (ed). Symposium on continuing care of the high-risk infant. Clin Perinatol 1984;11(1):1–244

Philipson EH, Kalham SC, Riha MM, Pimentel R. Effects of maternal glucose infusion on fetal acid–base status in human pregnancy. Am J Obstet Gynecol 1987;157(4):866–873

Thompson JE, Clark DA, Salisbury B, Cahill J. Footprinting the newborn infant: not cost effective. J Pediatr 1981;99(5):797–798

CHAPTER 5

PERINATAL INFECTIONS

Certain infections that occur antepartum or intrapartum may have a significant effect on the fetus and newborn; proper management of the mother during pregnancy and at delivery and of the newborn postnatally can prevent or modify many serious problems and can minimize the risk of subsequent transmission of infection in the nursery. Although many infections can have such an impact, those discussed here have been selected on the basis of new and evolving information that affects management. Close communication and cooperation among all perinatal care personnel are essential to obtain the best results.

There is no value to routine serologic screening for toxoplasmosis, cytomegalovirus (CMV), and herpes. Testing for these infections should be limited to patients in whom specific exposure is suspected. Therefore, TORCH (toxoplasmosis, other viruses, rubella, CMV, herpes simplex viruses) screening as a package is inappropriate.

Viral Infections

Cytomegalovirus Infection

Of women susceptible to CMV, the risk of primary infection during pregnancy is approximately 1% of live births. Primary CMV infections during pregnancy are usually asymptomatic, but the probability of intrauterine transmission of infection to the fetus is approximately 50%. Only 5–10% of these congenitally infected infants have clinically apparent disease; of those who do, however, the mortality ranges from 20–30%, and more than 90% of survivors develop significant sequelae. Of the congenitally infected infants who do not have clinically apparent infection as newborns, 10% develop late complications or sequelae, with sensorineural hearing loss being the most common. In general, the risk of neonatal disease with subsequent complications is higher if the mother has a primary CMV infection during the first half of pregnancy.

No specific recommendations can be made to prevent CMV infections of pregnant women. Routine serologic screening of pregnant women is not recommended because there is no reliable way to determine whether intrauterine infection or fetal disease has occurred, and the incidence is very low.

Neonates of seronegative mothers are at risk of severe morbidity or death if they acquire CMV infection. Although the risk of congenital CMV infection is lower in seropositive mothers, perinatal infection can occur. These infections can be transmitted to neonates by transfusion of blood from seropositive donors or by ingestion of CMV-contaminated milk from human milk banks. Transmission of CMV by these routes can be virtually eliminated by the use of blood or milk from CMV-negative donors or of frozen deglycerolized red blood cells by removal of the buffy coat or by filtration to remove the white blood cells. The use of CMV hyperimmune globulin is under investigation.

Hepatitis B Virus Infection

Maternal Infection

The Centers for Disease Control has recommended that hepatitis B vaccine be administered to all infants, including those born to hepatitis B surface antigen (HBsAg)-negative mothers. The recommended doses and schedule for administration of hepatitis B vaccine are shown in Tables 5-1 and 5-2.

In a pregnant woman, hepatitis B virus (HBV) infection may result in severe disease for the mother and chronic infection for the newborn, including chronic hepatitis, cirrhosis, and primary hepatocellular carcinoma. Although intrauterine infection may occur, transmission of HBV from mother to neonate apparently occurs most often during delivery. Neonates born to mothers who are infected with HBV during the last trimester of pregnancy are at high risk (approximately 80%) of acquiring infection. Neonates born to mothers who are chronic carriers of HBsAg are also at risk of developing infection. Because of the susceptibility of neonates to HBV infection and the high probability that those infected will develop chronic disease, it is important to identify pregnant women who are chronic HBsAg carriers. Studies have shown that historical information about risk factors reveals only a portion of women who are chronic carriers. Therefore, the test for HBsAg should be added to the battery of routine prenatal tests (no other test for hepatitis B screening is needed). If the patient has not been tested, the test should be performed on admission to the hospital. Once pregnant women who are chronic HBsAg carriers have been identified, prophylactic treatment with hepatitis B immune globulin (HBIg) and hepatitis B vaccine can be provided for their newborns. Prophylaxis for exposed newborns given within the first 24 hours is 85–95% effective in preventing neonatal infection and, probably, the frequency of the potentially life-threatening sequelae.

Women who are HBsAg negative but who have a history placing them at continuing high risk of HBV infection should be counseled about the advisability of vaccination. The adult dosage is 1 ml injected in the deltoid muscle; intramuscular injection in the buttocks is not as effective. A series of three doses is required; the second and third doses are given 1 and 6 months, respectively, after the first. Pregnancy is not a contraindication to vaccination.

Household contacts and sexual partners of HBsAg-positive women identified through prenatal screening should be vaccinated after testing to determine susceptibility to HBV infection when feasible. Hepatitis B vaccine should be given at the age-appropriate dose to those determined to be susceptible or judged likely to be susceptible to hepatitis B infection.

Management of Newborns Exposed to HBV

Neonates born to mothers who are HBsAg positive should receive the appropriate dose of hepatitis B vaccine and HBIg intramuscularly once they are physiologically stable, preferably within 12 hours of age (see Tables 5-1 and 5-2). They should be given concurrently, but at a different site. In order to avoid inoculation of virus contaminating the skin, the injection site should be cleaned. In addition, infants should receive subsequent doses of vaccine to complete the appropriate hepatitis B vaccine series. Data on the effectiveness of hepatitis B vaccine for neonates who weigh less than 2,000 g at birth are not available; however, the same

Table 5-1. Recommended Doses*

Infants of†	Recombivax HB	Engerix-B
HBsAg-positive mothers	5 µg (0.5 ml)	10 µg (0.5 ml)
HBsAg-negative mothers	2.5 µg (0.25 ml)	10 µg (0.5 ml)

*Usual schedule of three doses for both vaccines given at 0, 1, and 6 months; Engerix-B alternative schedule for four doses at 0, 1, 2, and 12 months.

†HBsAg, Hepatitis B surface antigen.

Table modified from Centers for Disease Control. Hepatitis B virus: a comprehensive strategy for eliminating transmission in the United States through universal childhood vaccination: recommendations of the Immunization Practices Advisory Committee (ACIP). MMWR 1991;40 (RR-13):1–25 prophylactic treatment is recommended as for any other newborn. Infants of HBsAg-positive mothers should be tested at 9 months or later (1 month or more after the third dose) for HBsAg and antibodies to HBV to determine the outcome of immunoprophylaxis.

Infants of mothers with unknown HBsAg status should be administered hepatitis B vaccine within 12 hours of birth at a dose appropriate for infants born to HBsAg-positive mothers. If the mother is subsequently found to be positive, HBIg should be administered as soon as possible and within 7 days of birth, although the efficacy of HBIg after 48 hours of birth is unknown. If HBIg has not been given, it is important that the infant receive the second dose of hepatitis B vaccine at 1 month and not later than 2 months of age, because of the higher risk of infection. The last dose should be given at 6 months. If the mother is found to be negative, the infant should continue to receive hepatitis B vaccine as part of the routine immunization schedule using the dose appropriate for infants born to an HBsAg-negative mother.

Table 5-2. Recommended Schedule for Hepatitis B Vaccine

Infants of*	Dose†	Age
HBsAg-positive mothers	HB Vaccine 1	Birth–within 12 h
	HBIg (0.5 ml IM)	Birth–within 12 h
	HB Vaccine 2	1 mo
	HB Vaccine 3	6 mo
HBsAg-unknown mothers	HB Vaccine 1	Birth–within 12 h
	HBIg	If mother HBsAg positive, give 0.5 ml IM as soon as possible, *not* later than 1 wk after birth
	HB Vaccine 2	1–2 mo
	HB Vaccine 3	6 mo
HBsAg-negative mothers‡	HB Vaccine 1	Birth–within 12 h
	HB Vaccine 2	1–2 mo
	HB Vaccine 3	6–18 mo

*HBsAg, Hepatitis B surface antigen.

†HB, Hepatitis B; HBIg, hepatitis B immune globulin; IM, intramuscularly.

‡A second option is to administer HBV at 2-month intervals to conform to the schedules of other childhood vaccines, which can be administered concurrently.

Table modified from Centers for Disease Control. Hepatitis B virus: a comprehensive strategy for eliminating transmission in the United States through universal childhood vaccination: recommendations of the Immunization Practices Advisory Committee (ACIP). MMWR 1991;40 (RR-13):1–25

Herpes Simplex Virus Infection

Treatment and Counseling During Pregnancy

Patients who deliver vaginally with an active genital herpes simplex virus (HSV) lesion have a 50% risk of transmitting the infection to the neonate if the disease is primary and 0–8% risk if recurrent. However, most (70%) newborns infected with HSV are delivered of women who have neither active genital herpes nor a history of these lesions.

The safety of administering acyclovir systemically for the treatment of HSV-infected pregnant women has not yet been established; however, current data have not revealed any adverse effects on the fetus. Prophylactic administration of antiviral drugs to women with genital HSV infection at delivery is not presently indicated. However, in the presence of life-threatening HSV infection (eg, disseminated infection that includes encephalitis, pneumonitis, and hepatitis), acyclovir administered intravenously is probably of value. Among pregnant women without life-threatening disease, systemic acyclovir treatment is not currently recommended. The results of ongoing trials are pending.

Couples should be educated about the natural history of genital HSV infection and should be advised that, if only one partner is infected, they should abstain from sexual contact while lesions are present. Some consultants also recommend that asymptomatic HSV-infected persons use condoms in an attempt to minimize the risk of transmitting the infection to their partners. Pregnant women should be advised that it is particularly important to avoid sexual contact during the last several months of gestation if their partners have an active genital HSV infection.

Obstetric Management

Patients with a history of genital herpes should have a careful perineal examination at the time of delivery. If a lesion is present, a cesarean delivery should be performed. Weekly cervical and vaginal herpes screenings in asymptomatic women have not been shown to be predictive of newborn infection and therefore are not recommended. Once membranes have ruptured near term, delivery should be expedited if lesions are present. It may be advisable to avoid scalp electrodes in patients with a history of genital herpes. Patients with nongenital lesions may deliver vaginally if the lesion can be covered and draped away from the perineum.

Women with clinically evident genital or nongenital HSV infection can be managed safely with drainage/secretion precautions in the labor, delivery, and postpartum care areas. Those with primary lesions should be managed with contact isolation in private rooms. Health care personnel and the patient herself should use gloves for direct contact with the infected area or with contaminated dressings, and meticulous hand-washing is essential. Labor and delivery rooms require only routine, careful cleaning and disinfection before being used by another patient.

Management of Exposed Newborns

The incidence of neonatal HSV infection is low; estimates range from 1/3,000–1/20,000 live births. Most infants who develop HSV infection acquire their infection perinatally from their mothers. Most frequently, HSV infects a neonate during passage through the infected maternal lower genital tract, or it ascends to the fetus, sometimes even though membranes are apparently intact. Less common sources of neonatal infection include 1) postnatal transmission from the mother or father, most often from a nongenital infection (eg, mouth, hands, or around the breasts), and 2) postnatal transmission in the nursery from another infected neonate, probably on the hands of personnel attending the infants. Postnatal transmission from personnel with fever blisters to neonates appears to occur extremely rarely, if at all. Congenital (intrauterine) infection also occurs rarely.

Patterns of HSV infection in newborns are 1) a generalized, systemic infection including the liver, the central nervous system, and other organs; 2) localized central nervous system disease; or 3) localized infection of the skin, eyes, or mouth; or a combination of 1–3. Clinical onset of disease usually occurs during the first month. Disseminated disease usually occurs during the first 1–2 weeks of life; disease localized to the central nervous system or to the skin, eyes, or mouth more often occurs during the second or third week. Approximately one third of neonates with HSV infection develop lesions of the skin, eyes, or mouth as an early manifestation; in another one third, there may be other evidence of systemic or central nervous system disease before the mucocutaneous lesions appear; and in one third, there are no visible lesions. Asymptomatic HSV infection of newborns occurs rarely, if at all.

Nursery Management. Precautions should be taken to minimize the risk of transmission within the nursery. Neonates with documented perinatal exposure to HSV may be in the incubation phase of infection and should be handled expectantly. Neonates born vaginally (or by cesarean delivery if membranes had ruptured) to a mother with active HSV lesions should be managed with contact isolation if they remain in the nursery during the incubation period; an isolation room is not essential. An alternative approach is to have the neonate stay with the mother in a private room after instructing the mother regarding proper preventive care to reduce postpartum transmission. Personnel working with these potentially infected neonates should wash their hands meticulously after caring for the neonates.

The risk of HSV infection in neonates (eg, those born to an asymptomatic mother with a history of recurrent genital herpes or born to a symptomatic mother by cesarean delivery before rupture of membranes) is extremely low. Special isolation precautions are not needed for most of these neonates. They should be observed for several days and followed closely after discharge, however, and their parents should be instructed to observe them carefully for early signs of infection.

Early Diagnosis and Management. Early signs of HSV infection in newborns are frequently nonspecific and subtle. A neonate known to have been exposed to HSV should be observed carefully for vesicular lesions or for unexplained illnesses, including respiratory distress, convulsions, or signs of sepsis. If any of these occur, the possibility of HSV infection should be investigated. Skin lesions and other sites, as appropriate, should be cultured for HSV. The neonate should be physically segregated and managed with contact isolation; an isolation room is desirable. Personnel having contact with skin lesions or potentially infectious secretions should use gowns and gloves. Antiviral therapy should be initiated if HSV is strongly suspected; expert consultation about recommended antiviral drug therapy should be sought. Neonates with HSV disease should be managed in a facility that provides level III care.

Cultures obtained from the nasopharynx or mouth and the conjunctivae of neonates born to mothers known to be, or strongly suspected of being, infected with HSV can assist in management decisions. Cultures obtained from the neonate shortly after birth are helpful in identifying exposed neonates, but they do not indicate HSV infection. Furthermore, the sensitivity of these cultures in predicting infection is unknown. A positive culture obtained 24–48 hours or longer after birth suggests HSV infection and is an indication for immediate institution of antiviral therapy, even in the absence of symptoms.

Although HSV infection is more likely to occur at a site of skin trauma, there are no data to indicate that the circumcision of male neonates who may have been exposed at birth should be postponed. Delay of circumcision for approximately 1 month for those neonates at highest risk of disease (eg, those born vaginally to mothers with active genital lesions) may be prudent, however.

Contact of Neonates with Their HSV-Infected Mothers

A mother with HSV infection should be taught about her infection and hygienic measures to prevent postpartum transmission of the infection to her neonate. Before touching her newborn, the mother should wash her hands carefully and don a clean gown or use a clean barrier to ensure that the neonate does not come into contact with lesions or potentially infectious material. If the mother has genital herpes infection, her newborn may room-in with her after she has been taught protective measures. Breast-feeding is permissible if the mother has no vesicular herpetic lesions in the breast area and all active cutaneous lesions are covered.

A mother with herpes labialis (cold sore) or stomatitis should not kiss or nuzzle her newborn until the lesions have cleared. She may wear a disposable surgical mask when she touches her newborn until the lesions have crusted and dried. Herpetic lesions on other skin sites should be covered. Direct contact of a newborn with other family members or friends who have active HSV infection should be avoided.

Human Immune Deficiency Virus Infection

In the United States, the prevalence of human immune deficiency virus (HIV) infection in women of childbearing age is approximately 1.5/1,000. Seroprevalence data from newborn heel stick specimens indicate wide geographic variation. Seroprevalence is highest in metropolitan areas, but it is increasing in small (population 50,000–100,000) urban and rural areas.

HIV may be present in the blood and semen or vaginal and cervical secretions of infected persons. The primary means of transmission have been sexual contact and shared use of blood-contaminated needles and syringes in intravenous drug abuse. The end stage of infection with HIV is acquired immune deficiency syndrome (AIDS).

The reported cases of AIDS in women indicate that women are most likely to be infected through intravenous drug abuse (52%), sexual contact with a man known to be at risk of HIV infection (31%), and blood transfusions or clotting factor therapy given before mid-1985 (10%), when programs to screen blood for HIV began. The significance of intravenous drug abuse in the transmission of HIV to women is magnified by the fact that most of the heterosexually transmitted infections occurred from sexual contact with a man infected through drug abuse.

The risk of congenital (intrauterine, presumably transplacental) or intrapartum transmission of HIV from an infected woman to her fetus or newborn depends on multiple factors. The best estimates of vertical transmission of HIV from an infected woman range from 12.9–39%.

Cesarean delivery does not appear to protect the neonate from HIV infection.

Since HIV infection may occasionally be transmitted to infants through breast-feeding, breast-feeding should be discouraged in HIV-infected women when safe alternative feedings are available. Other types of postpartum transmission from a mother to her newborn (eg, through routine care and affection for the infant) have not been documented; the relative risk of this type of transmission appears to be very low.

Diagnosis

Adults and Children. Because persons infected with HIV usually develop antibody within 6–12 weeks of infection, the diagnosis of HIV infection in adults and older children is most often established through a validated serologic test for antibody. Screening tests based on enzyme immunoassay (EIA) or enzyme-linked immunosorbent assay (ELISA) are highly sensitive and specific when a serum specimen is found to give consistently reactive results. Because of the low prevalence of HIV infection in many populations, however, and because of the extraordinary social and medical implications of positive test results, the serum specimen from a person with a repeatedly reactive EIA or ELISA should also be tested by a supplemental or validation test. Currently, this is most often a Western blot test. Additional types of laboratory procedures for diagnosis of HIV infection will be available in the future.

Infants. Because of the transplacental passage of maternal HIV antibody to virtually all infants born to mothers who are infected, the diagnosis of HIV infection in newborns is extremely difficult with the laboratory methods currently available. The presence of HIV antibody as detected by EIA, ELISA, Western blot tests, or other methods should be expected in the serum of an infant born to a seropositive mother. An infant who is not infected should remain healthy, and the titer of antibody should decline during the first year; a few infants have not seroreverted until 15–18 months after birth. The loss of HIV antibody is not unequivocal evidence that the infant is free of infection, however, because a percentage of infants who serorevert are HIV infected, but appear to be immune tolerant. Infection of the infant is suggested when serial specimens assayed at one time by the same technique show persistent or rising titers of HIV antibody or when new HIV-specific antibody bands not present in the mother's serum appear on diagnostic tests such as Western blot or radio-immuno-precipitation assay. New diagnostic techniques currently being studied may permit earlier detection of infected infants.

Currently, definitive evidence of HIV infection in infants must be based on 1) a diagnosis of AIDS, 2) a combination of HIV antibody and a compatible immunologic profile and clinical course, or 3) detection of HIV in blood or tissues. Methods for detection of HIV in blood include virus culture, which is definitive if positive but is not highly sensitive; tests for HIV antigen, which will be widely available in the near future but do not yet have documented sensitivity and specificity in infants; and assay for viral nucleic acids, which is likely to be sensitive and specific but is still experimental.

Prevention

The only effective preventive measures involve avoiding contact with infected bodily fluids, such as blood, semen, and vaginal secretions. All pregnant women should be offered screening, and those who are in high seroprevalence areas (≥1/1,000) or believed to be at increased risk of HIV infection should be counseled and strongly urged to undergo testing for HIV antibody. The identification of an HIV-infected pregnant woman as early in pregnancy as possible is important to ensure appropriate counseling and medical care, including pregnancy termination if this is her choice; to plan medical care for the infant; and to provide counseling about family planning, future pregnancies, and the risk of sexual transmission of HIV to others. Testing should be done only after her informed consent is given. Many states have specific legal requirements concerning consent and confidentiality of HIV testing. Physicians should be aware of applicable laws and regulations in their states. Seroprevalence data for pregnant women can be obtained from Centers for Disease Control/state health department anonymous newborn screening programs.

Management

Because HIV (as well as other agents such as HBV) may be present in blood, vaginal secretions, and other fluids (eg, amniotic fluid), it is recommended that universal precautions should be followed for all vaginal and cesarean deliveries because many women with HIV infection may not be identified. Use of precautions only in women with known HIV infection is not optimal. Gloves should be used when handling the placenta or the neonate until blood and amniotic fluid have been removed from the neonate's skin. Fetal scalp electrodes should be avoided in HIV-positive women.

After delivery, women infected with HIV can be managed in the postpartum care unit with universal precautions. Appropriate medical follow-up for the mother should be arranged to minimize complications from her HIV infection.

Few infants with HIV infection show clinical evidence of infection in the first weeks after birth. In order to minimize the risk to health care personnel, all infants should be managed with universal precautions. Prompt and careful removal of blood from a neonate's skin is important. There is no need for other special precautions or for isolation of the neonate with an HIV-infected mother; rooming-in is acceptable. Gloves should be worn for contact with blood or blood-containing fluids and for procedures that involve exposure to blood. Gloves are not required for prevention of HIV transmission while changing diapers in usual circumstances.

The potential for HIV infection in neonates whose mothers are infected should be kept in mind and diagnostic procedures requested as appropriate and available. Because potentially HIV-infected infants have special diagnostic and care needs, arrangements for appropriate pediatric care should be made before these infants are discharged from the hospital.

Human Papillomavirus Infection

Genital warts caused by human papillomavirus (HPV) are becoming more common. Infection with HPV also appears to be related to the subsequent development of genital neoplasms. Cervical or vaginal HPV infections are usually asymptomatic, and Pap tests are useful for the diagnosis of subclinical cervical infection. Most genital HPV infections are sexually transmitted.

Genital HPV infections may exacerbate during pregnancy. The papillary lesions may proliferate on the vulva and in the vagina, and lesions may become increasingly friable during pregnancy. For the treatment of genital HPV infection in pregnancy, cryotherapy, laser therapy, and trichloroacetic acid may be used safely. Podophyllin, 5-fluorouracil, and interferon should not be used during pregnancy for removal of large lesions in the vagina or vulva.

There is a small risk that an infant whose mother has a genital HPV infection will develop subsequent respiratory papillomatosis. These lesions are now known to be caused by HPV types 6 and 11. Possible modes of transmission include contact between the fetus and the infected genital tract of the mother, transplacental passage of maternal infection, or postnatal contact with an infected individual. There is usually a latent period of years before HPV lesions become clinically significant in children. Because the risk of respiratory papillomatosis is low, cesarean delivery is not recommended solely to protect the neonate from HPV infection. However, cesarean delivery may be necessary in women who have extensive condylomata because of poor vulvar distensibility. Neonates born to mothers with HPV infection do not need to be managed with special precautions in the nursery.

Human Parvovirus Infection

The agent of erythema infectiosum is a single-stranded DNA virus called parvovirus B19, which infects humans only. When maternal parvovirus B19 infection occurs in pregnancy, the fetus is usually not affected. Well-documented cases of fetal hydrops and death following parvovirus B19 infection of the mother have been reported, however. The virus infects erythroid precursors, causing fetal anemia and leading to hydrops and death. Most reported maternal infections that have resulted in fetal death occurred in the first half of the pregnancy, with fetal death and spontaneous abortion usually taking place 4–6 weeks after infection. Third-trimester maternal infections followed by the birth of anemic newborns were recently described. A parvovirus-associated fetal anomaly has not yet been established. Thus far it appears that infection during pregnancy can be embryocidal, but, if not, teratogenic effects are absent.

Parvovirus infection is an infrequent cause of spontaneous abortion; it was responsible for less than 1% of spontaneous abortions in one study. Based on the limited data available, about 50% of women in an average American city will be immune to parvovirus B19. The risk of fetal death to a woman exposed occupationally would usually be much less than 1%.

Pregnant women who subsequently find they have been in contact with children who are in the incubation period of erythema infectiosum or children who are in aplastic crisis should have the relatively low potential risk explained to them. The contagious period occurs before the rash appears, thus the infection is not contagious at the time of eruption. Fetal ultrasound determinations may be useful in detecting hydrops. Women who are exposed to children at work (such as teachers or day care workers) or at home are at increased risk of infection with parvovirus B19. However, because of widespread inapparent infection in both adults and children, all women are at some risk of exposure, particularly those women with school-aged children. In view of the high prevalence of parvovirus B19, the low risk of ill effect to the fetus, and the fact that avoidance of child care or teaching can only reduce but not eliminate the risk of infection, a policy of routinely excluding pregnant women from the work place where erythema infectiosum is present is not recommended. However, pregnant health care workers should not care for patients with aplastic crisis, who may be highly contagious.

Rubella

Prevention and Management During Pregnancy

Surveillance for susceptibility to rubella infection is essential in prenatal care. Each patient should be screened serologically at the first prenatal visit unless she is proved to be immune by a previous serologic test. In a properly controlled test, any detectable antibody indicates immunity.

Seropositive women do not need further testing, regardless of their subsequent history of exposure. If seronegative pregnant women have been exposed to rubella or develop symptoms that suggest infection, however, their antibody titers should be repeated to determine whether infection occurred. Specimens should be obtained soon as possible after exposure, 2 weeks later, and, if necessary, 4 weeks after exposure. Serum specimens from both acute and convalescent periods should be tested on the same day in the same laboratory; a fourfold or greater rise in titer or seroconversion indicates acute infection. Rubella-specific immunoglobulin M testing or isolation of the virus from throat swabs rapidly establishes a diagnosis of acute rubella if the tests are available.

If rubella is diagnosed in a pregnant woman, the patient should be advised of the risks of fetal infection, and the alternative of therapeutic abortion should be discussed. Limited data indicate that the administration of immune globulin, 0.55 ml/kg, as soon as possible after exposure may prevent or modify infection in exposed susceptible persons, but there are no data to show that immune globulin prevents fetal infection. The absence of clinical signs in a woman who has received immune globulin does not guarantee that infection has been prevented, however; neonates with congenital rubella syndrome have been born to mothers given immune globulin shortly after exposure. If a woman chooses not to terminate her pregnancy, administration of immune globulin as soon as possible after exposure should be considered.

For rubella-susceptible women of reproductive age, the vaccine is highly effective and has few side effects. The puerperium is an excellent time to vaccinate susceptible women. Prevaccination serologic testing for susceptibility is not mandatory and should not impede vaccination, but serum may be tested 6–8 weeks postvaccination to confirm seroconversion.

Vaccinated women, including those vaccinated during the puerperium, should be warned to avoid conception for 3 months because of the theoretical risk that vaccine virus could be teratogenic, even though the risk of fetal infection with the current vaccine is less than 3%. A woman who conceives within 3 months of rubella vaccination or who is inadvertently vaccinated in early pregnancy should be counseled that the risks to the fetus are theoretical and that data do not support an assumption that the pregnancy should be terminated. At present, no case of rubella syndrome has arisen from a mother given human diploid vaccine RA 27/3. To assist in the development of firm recommendations for the management of this problem, physicians caring for a susceptible pregnant woman inadvertently immunized with rubella vaccine within 3 months before or after conception should report the case as soon as possible to the Division of Immunization, Centers for Disease Control.

Management of Neonates

Neonates who show signs of congenital rubella infection or who were born to women known to have had rubella during pregnancy should be managed with contact isolation, preferably in a private room. Care should be provided only by personnel known to be immune to rubella. Every effort should be made to isolate the virus from the neonate and to document the infection. Neonates with congenital rubella should be considered contagious up to 1 year of age unless viral cultures are negative. Cases of congenital rubella syndrome or birth defects believed to be caused by rubella infection should be reported to the state health department.

Varicella-Zoster Virus Infection

Women with varicella-zoster virus infection (chickenpox) during pregnancy are no more likely to develop varicella pneumonia than are other adults, but varicella pneumonia is more severe in pregnancy. Thus, pregnant women with varicella should be followed closely for pulmonary symptoms. There is no evidence that maternal administration of varicella-zoster immune globulin (VZIg) reduces the rare occurrence of congenital varicella syndrome. However, routine passive immunization probably ameliorates the illness in nonimmune pregnant women as in other adults. Thus, a woman who has been exposed to varicella (through intimate or household contact) and who has no history of prior infection should be tested for immunity. If she is not immune, VZIg should be administered. VZIg is available from the American Red Cross Blood Services. Varicella during early pregnancy is rarely associated with severe congenital malformations or fetal mortality. If onset of clinical maternal infection occurs within 4–5 days of delivery (ie, prior to the maternal antibody response), subsequent infection in the newborn may be fulminant, with systemic and neurologic involvement and death. In such cases, VZIg should be administered directly to the neonate as soon as possible after delivery. Once

VZIg is administered, the neonate can be with the mother. Likewise, when maternal varicella infection is diagnosed within 2 days following delivery, VZIg is indicated for the neonate. VZIg administered to the mother within 4–5 days prior to delivery is unlikely to reach the fetus in sufficient quantities.

Women with varicella must be kept in strict isolation if admitted to a hospital. Neonates exposed in utero or postnatally to varicella should be segregated and managed expectantly during the incubation period. Those neonates with varicella infection should be isolated in a private room and managed with strict isolation for the duration of illness. Neonates with congenital varicella acquired earlier in gestation do not need to be managed with special precautions.

Very premature infants (less than 28 weeks of gestation) who are exposed postnatally should receive VZIg (125 U) because of poor transfer of antibody across the placenta early in pregnancy.

Bacterial Infections

Group B Streptococcal Infection

The proportion of pregnant women colonized with group B streptococci (GBS) ranges from approximately 5–35% but may be intermittent. Group B streptococci account for significant postpartum infection (eg, endometritis, amnionitis, and urinary tract infections), but antepartum rectal or genital colonization is asymptomatic.

Infection frequently is transmitted from the mother to the newborn, either in utero or intrapartum; nosocomial neonatal infection (probably neonate to neonate via the hands of personnel) also occurs. Group B streptococci are important causes of disease in the neonate and infant. Neonatal group B streptococcal disease has an incidence of 1–5 cases per 1,000 live births. Early-onset disease occurs in approximately 1% of infants born to colonized women. The risk of early-onset disease is increased by low birth weight, prolonged interval between rupture of amniotic membranes and delivery (greater than 12–18 hours), and clinically evident amnionitis. Low (or absent) levels of type-specific serum GBS antibody also may predispose neonates to disease.

Routine prenatal cultures to detect colonization are not recommended because 1) colonization may be intermittent; 2) the predictive value of a single genital culture in the prenatal period is only 60–70% for a positive culture at delivery; and 3) with a low attack rate (about 1%), there is a large expense. However, the administration of ampicillin during labor to colonized women with high-risk factors (eg, premature labor, prolonged rupture of membranes, or maternal fever) has been shown to decrease infection significantly in their infants. Thus, it is appropriate to perform a genital culture for GBS in patients who are admitted with premature labor or premature rupture of membranes, or who develop fever in labor. Since presumptive identification of GBS can be made in the laboratory, usually within 24–48 hours, the culture will be available before most of these patients at risk are likely to deliver. For the patient who is at risk of delivering before the GBS culture is available, some clinicians advocate empiric selective intrapartum antibiotics to ensure that those who are colonized receive this regimen. Without culture results, the risk to the mother and her infant from the emergence of ampicillin-resistant organisms is unknown. Furthermore, preliminary data suggest that the intrapartum administration of ampicillin to women who have previously delivered infected neonates may be beneficial. Routinely obtaining specimens for culture to determine whether neonates have been colonized with GBS, either to identify those who could be treated or to control infection, is not recommended.

Neonates with group B streptococcal disease may be treated in the intensive care area if contact isolation precautions are taken to prevent the transmission of bacterial infection. Antibiotics are the mainstay of therapy. In view of the high percentage of colonized neonates within many nurseries and the lack of any effective means to eradicate colonization, routine identification and isolation of asymptomatic carriers are impractical. Other methods of control (eg, treatment of asymptomatic carriers with penicillin or treatment of the umbilical cord with triple dye or hexachlorophene) are impractical or unreliable for control of GBS.

Detection of nosocomial infection by GBS is difficult because most neonates have late-onset disease that may not appear until days or weeks after discharge from the nursery. If a cluster of cases occurs in neonates born at a single hospital, however, an investigation is warranted. Establishing cohorts of ill and colonized neonates in the nursery may be useful. Meticulous hand-washing by all personnel, sufficient personnel on all shifts, and adequate spacing between neonates may be important in limiting neonate-to-neonate transmission within the nursery.

Listeriosis

The epidemiology of infection with *Listeria monocytogenes* has remained obscure. It is believed that the fetus or newborn acquires *L. monocytogenes* most often through maternal bacteremia (transplacentally), through ascending maternal genital tract infection, or during birth; nosocomial transmission to newborns probably occurs as well. Signs of listeriosis in the newborn are highly variable and often nonspecific. The clinical picture may be similar to that of group B streptococcal infection with early- and late-onset syndromes. Early-onset listeriosis often resembles respiratory distress or heart failure; late-onset disease more often causes meningitis.

L. monocytogenes can be cultured readily, but the laboratory should be informed that this organism is suspected, as *L. monocytogenes* may be confused initially with lactobacilli. Special techniques may be necessary to isolate the organism from stool and other sites with mixed flora. Gram stain of a fecal smear from an infected newborn may show the organism in profusion.

Prompt diagnosis and antibiotic treatment of maternal listeriosis may prevent fetal or perinatal infection. *L. monocytogenes* is highly sensitive to penicillin/ampicillin. Because some women have had repeated fetal infection with *L. monocytogenes*, some authorities suggest that the cervix and stools of the mother of an infected infant be cultured and the mother treated if either culture is positive. Reculturing during a subsequent pregnancy has also been suggested, but the usefulness of this measure has not been evaluated.

Neonates with listeriosis should be managed in the nursery with drainage/secretion precautions.

Syphilis

The incidence of syphilis in the United States is increasing. Pregnant women should undergo serologic screening for syphilis at the first prenatal visit and after exposure to an infected partner. As false-negative screening tests may occur in early primary infection, another test for syphilis should be performed in the third trimester if the patient belongs to a high-risk population. The specificity of serologic testing is high if both a nontreponemal screening test and a subsequent treponemal serologic test are reactive. Dark-field and histologic examinations are the most reliable when lesions are present.

Congenital syphilis is most often acquired through hematogenous transplacental infection of the fetus, although direct contact of the neonate with infectious lesions during or after birth can also result in infection. Transplacental infection can occur throughout pregnancy and at any stage of maternal infection.

Pregnant women with syphilis should be treated with penicillin. If they are allergic to penicillin, they should be desensitized and then treated with penicillin. One regimen suggested for desensitization is shown in

Table 5-3. Oral Desensitization Protocol

Dose*	Penicillin V Suspension (U/ml)	Amount† (ml)	Amount† (U)	Cumulative Dose (U)
1	1,000	0.1	100	100
2	1,000	0.2	200	300
3	1,000	0.4	400	700
4	1,000	0.8	800	1,500
5	1,000	1.6	1,600	3,100
6	1,000	3.2	3,200	6,300
7	1,000	6.4	6,400	12,700
8	10,000	1.2	12,000	24,700
9	10,000	2.4	24,000	48,700
10	10,000	4.8	48,000	96,700
11	80,000	1.0	80,000	176,700
12	80,000	2.0	160,000	336,700
13	80,000	4.0	320,000	656,700
14	80,000	8.0	640,000	1,296,700

Observation period: 30 minutes before parenteral administration of penicillin.

*Interval between doses, 15 minutes; elapsed time, 3 hours and 45 minutes; cumulative dose, 1.3 million U.

†The specific amount of drug was diluted in approximately 30 ml of water and then given orally.

Adapted with permission from Wendel GD Jr, Stark BJ, Jamison RB, Molina RD, Sullivan TJ. Penicillin allergy and desensitization in serious infections during pregnancy. N Engl J Med 1985;312:1229–1232

Table 5-3. Tetracycline and doxycycline are contraindicated in pregnancy. Erythromycin should not be used because of the high risk of failure to cure infection in the fetus.

The results of the maternal serologic tests and treatment, if given, should be recorded in the neonate's medical record or be made available to the neonate's physician. A serologic test for syphilis should be performed on cord or venous blood of neonates for whom the results of maternal tests or treatment are unavailable or questionable.

A diagnosis of congenital syphilis is frequently difficult to establish because clinical evidence of infection may not be apparent at birth and the results of serologic tests may be equivocal. Neonates with a positive result on a serologic test for syphilis or a history of partial or questionably adequate maternal treatment for infection must be followed carefully. A reactive serologic test for syphilis (eg, Venereal Disease Research Laboratory or fluorescent treponemal antibody absorption [FTA-ABS] test) on cord or neonatal blood does not necessarily indicate that the neonate is infected. If the reaction is caused only by passively transferred antibody, the Venereal Disease Research Laboratory titer is usually lower than the mother's and reverts to negative in 4–6 months. A positive result on the FTA-ABS test caused by passively transferred antibody may take as long as 1 year to become negative. A persistently reactive serologic test for syphilis suggests infection, and a rising titer is almost diagnostic. The immunoglobulin M FTA-ABS test is not totally specific; because false-negative results may be obtained, a negative test result does not exclude active infection in the neonate.

Clinical symptoms of early congenital syphilis may be nonspecific. Long bone roentgenograms may be useful in establishing a diagnosis. The cerebrospinal fluid of infants with suspected or proven congenital syphilis should be examined for evidence of neurosyphilis.

Moist, open syphilitic lesions are infectious. Drainage/secretion precautions and blood/body fluid precautions should be used when it is suspected that a neonate has congenital syphilis. Health care personnel (and parents) should wear gloves when handling the neonate until appropriate antibiotic therapy has been administered for 24 hours. Individuals who had close contact with the neonate before isolation precautions and treatment were instituted should be examined clinically and tested serologically for infection.

Treatment of neonates with congenital syphilis is summarized in Table 5-4. For further information, refer to *Report of the Committee on Infectious Diseases*, 22nd edition, published by the American Academy of Pediatrics.

Lyme Disease

The epidemiology of Lyme disease began with the observation of a marked increase in juvenile arthritis in Lyme, Connecticut. It was then determined that this epidemic was caused by *Borrelia burgdorferi*, a spirochete transmitted by ticks (*Ixodes dammini* or related *Ixodes* ticks). In the western United States, the disease may be transmitted by *Ixodes pacificus*. Early stages of this illness, which now has been reported nationally, are characterized by a distinctive bull's-eye skin lesion (erythema migrans), which is seen is 60–80% of patients, and nonspecific flulike symptoms. Untreated disease may result in neurologic or cardiac manifestations, which may appear within 4–6 weeks after the onset of early signs and symptoms. A late manifestation of Lyme disease is arthritis, usually intermittent inflammatory arthritis of a large joint. Approximately 60% of untreated patients will develop joint involvement ranging from mild to moderate arthralgia to chronic destructive joint disease.

Table 5-4. Recommended Treatment of Congenital Syphilis

Clinical Status	Antibiotic Therapy*
Proved or highly probable disease	
Age	
≤ 4 wks	Aqueous crystalline penicillin G, IV or IM, for 10–14 d[†]
> 4 wks	Aqueous crystalline penicillin G, IV or IM, for 10–14 d[†]
Asymptomatic infant with normal cerebrospinal fluid and radiographic examinations	
Maternal Treatment	
None, inadequate, undocumented, or with erythromycin	Aqueous crystalline penicillin G, IV or IM, for 10 d[†],[§]
Adequate therapy given in last month before delivery	Aqueous crystalline penicillin G, IV or IM, for 10 d[†] or benzathine penicillin G, IM, single dose
Adequate therapy given > 1 mo before delivery	Clinical and serologic follow-up only, or if follow-up cannot be ensured, benzathine penicillin G, IM, single dose, or aqueous crystalline penicillin G, IV or IM, for 10 d[†]

*IV, intravenously; IM, intramuscularly.

[†]Some experts recommend aqueous procaine penicillin G, IM, for 10–14 days.

[‡]For those with late (> 1 year of age) congenital syphilis in whom cerebrospinal fluid findings exclude neurosyphilis, some experts recommend benzathine penicillin G IM weekly for 3 weeks.

[§]Alternatively, for the infant for whom adequate maternal treatment cannot be documented, some experts recommend single-dose therapy with benzathine penicillin G.

From American Academy of Pediatrics, Committee on Infectious Diseases. Report of the committee on infectious diseases. 22nd ed. Elk Grove village, IL: AAP, 1991

There are no definitive early diagnostic tests. In early stages of the illness, only 50% or fewer patients will have a seropositive ELISA or indirect fluorescent antibody test for *B. burgdorferi*. Patients with late Lyme disease will usually be seropositive. Suspicion of early maternal infection is based on a history of exposure to tick bites, the presence of the distinctive skin lesion, and nonspecific flulike symptoms. Since the presence of erythema migrans is diagnostic, it may be helpful to enlist the aid of an experienced physician to examine the woman.

Spirochetes cross the placenta and have been found in the tissues of stillborn fetuses; however, the frequency of fetal infection is unknown. Hence, the obstetric dilemma is when to treat women suspected of having early-onset Lyme disease but who have a negative serology. It may be preferable to treat pregnant patients on the basis of the described clinical picture prior to the development of late maternal disease. Current data do not support counseling for pregnancy termination.

Adequate prophylactic therapy for deer tick bites during pregnancy or treatment of suspected early disease would be 3 weeks of either amoxicillin, 500 mg three times daily, or penicillin V, 500 mg four times daily. Erythromycin at a dose of 250–500 mg four times daily has been reported to be less effective, but it is the secondary choice for pregnant women who are allergic to penicillin. Adequately treated patients may never develop antibodies to spirochetes.

The infant's health care provider should be informed when maternal disease is suspected. The decision of whether to treat the newborn of a woman with suspected or proven Lyme disease should be discussed with the attendant pediatrician.

The best preventive measure is to avoid heavily wooded areas. If entrance into such areas is necessary, it is best to wear long-sleeved shirts and long pants tucked in at the ankle.

Chlamydial Infection

Chlamydia trachomatis has been generally detected in the cervix of approximately 2–13% of pregnant women, but the prevalence is as high as 25% in selected populations. The prevalence tends to be highest in young women (< age 20 years) and in those with a history of other sexually transmitted diseases. Most infected women are asymptomatic, but *Chlamydia* may cause urethritis and mucopurulent (nongonococcal) cervicitis. Chlamydial infection is also associated with postpartum endometritis and infertility. Infection may be transmitted from the genital tract of infected mothers to their neonates during birth; 60–70% of neonates born to infected mothers without prophylaxis acquire *C. trachomatis*. Purulent conjunctivitis occurs in approximately 30–50% of neonates born vaginally to women with chlamydial infection, and neonatal pneumonia occurs in 10–20%.

Important risk factors for chlamydial infection include single marital status, age younger than 20 years, residence in a socially disadvantaged community (eg, inner city), history or presence of other sexually transmitted diseases, and little or no prenatal care. However, routine screening of all pregnant women for *C. trachomatis* is not recommended.

Treatment should be administered to women with known *C. trachomatis* infection (ie, with mucopurulent cervicitis) and to women whose sexual partners have nongonococcal urethritis and who are presumed to be infected when diagnostic tests are not performed. Erythromycin base is the drug of choice (500 mg four times daily for 10 days is effective;

alternatively, erythromycin base, 250 mg four times daily for 14 days). Simultaneous treatment of the male partner or partners with tetracycline or doxycycline is an important component of the therapeutic regimen.

Chlamydial infections in the neonate are generally mild and responsive to antimicrobial therapy; prophylactic cesarean delivery is not warranted. Prophylactic instillation of topical erythromycin or tetracycline into the conjunctival sac of the neonate shortly after birth helps to prevent inclusion conjunctivitis. The effectiveness of 0.5% erythromycin ophthalmologic ointment in the prevention of chlamydial conjunctivitis in one study has not been confirmed in subsequent studies. *C. trachomatis* also is susceptible to tetracyclines, but studies of clinical efficacy of tetracycline ointment in the prophylaxis of chlamydial conjunctivitis have also given conflicting results. Neither erythromycin nor tetracycline prevents chlamydial pneumonia. Neonates with inclusion conjunctivitis should be managed with drainage/secretion precautions. Those with chlamydial pneumonia should be managed similarly, and they should also be separated from neonates who are uninfected and neonates who are infected with other respiratory agents. Transmission of chlamydial infections within nurseries has been suspected, but not proved.

Resources and Recommended Reading

Advisory Committee on Immunization Practices. A comprehensive strategy for the elimination of hepatitis B virus transmission in the United States through universal childhood immunization. MMWR, in preparation

Advisory Committee on Immunization Practices. Prevention of perinatal transmission of hepatitis B virus. MMWR 1988;37:341–346, 351

American Academy of Pediatrics, Committee on Infectious Diseases. Parvovirus, erythema infectiosum and pregnancy. Pediatrics 1990;85:131–133

American Academy of Pediatrics, Committee on Infectious Diseases. Report of the committee on infectious diseases. 22nd ed. Elk Grove Village, IL: AAP, 1991

American Academy of Pediatrics, Task Force on Pediatric AIDS. Pediatric guidelines for infection control of human immunodeficiency virus (acquired immunodeficiency syndrome virus) in hospitals, medical offices, schools and other settings. Pediatrics 1988;82:801–807

American Academy of Pediatrics, Task Force on Pediatric AIDS. Perinatal human immunodeficiency virus infection. Pediatrics 1988;82:941–944

American College of Obstetricians and Gynecologists. Antimicrobial therapy for obstetric patients. ACOG Technical Bulletin 117. Washington, DC: ACOG, 1988

American College of Obstetricians and Gynecologists. Genital human papillomavirus infections. ACOG Technical Bulletin 105. Washington, DC: ACOG, 1987

American College of Obstetricians and Gynecologists. Gonorrhea and chlamydial infections. ACOG Technical Bulletin 89. Washington, DC: ACOG, 1985

American College of Obstetricians and Gynecologists. Guidelines for hepatitis B virus screening and vaccination during pregnancy. ACOG Committee Opinion 78. Washington, DC: ACOG, 1990

American College of Obstetricians and Gynecologists. Human immune deficiency virus infections. ACOG Technical Bulletin 123. Washington, DC: ACOG, 1988

American College of Obstetricians and Gynecologists. Perinatal herpes simplex virus infections. ACOG Technical Bulletin 122. Washington, DC: ACOG, 1988

American College of Obstetricians and Gynecologists. Perinatal viral and parasitic infections. ACOG Technical Bulletin 114. Washington, DC: ACOG, 1988

Arvin AM, Hensleigh PA, Prober CG, Au DS, Yasukawa LL, Wittek AE, et al. Failure of antepartum maternal cultures to predict the infants at risk of exposure to herpes simplex virus at delivery. N Engl J Med 1986;315:796–800

Boyer KM, Gotoff SP. Prevention of early-onset neonatal group B streptococcal disease with selective intrapartum chemoprophylaxis. N Engl J Med 1986;314:1665–1669

Brown ZA, Baker DA. Acyclovir therapy during pregnancy. Obstet Gynecol 1989;73:526–531

Brown ZA, Vontver LA, Benedetti J, Critchlow CW, Sells CJ, Berry S, et al. Effects on infants of a first episode of genital herpes during pregnancy. N Engl J Med 1987;317:1246–1251

Centers for Disease Control. 1989 sexually transmitted diseases treatment guidelines. MMWR 1989;38(8 suppl):5

Centers for Disease Control. Guidelines for prevention of transmission of human immunodeficiency virus and hepatitis B virus to health-care and public-safety workers. MMWR 1989;38(suppl 6):1–37

Centers for Disease Control. Risks associated with human parvovirus B19 infection. MMWR 1989;38:81–88, 93–97

Centers for Disease Control. Update: universal precautions for prevention of transmission of human immunodeficiency virus, hepatitis B virus, and other bloodborne pathogens in health-care settings. MMWR 1988;37:377–382, 387–388

Falloon J, Eddy J, Weiner L, Pizzo PA. Human immunodeficiency virus infection in children. J Pediatr 1989;1:1–30

Gibbs RS, Amstey MS, Sweet RL, Mead PB, Sever JL. Management of genital herpes infection. Obstet Gynecol 1988;71:779–780

Krivine A, Yakudima A, LeMay M, Pena-Cruz V, Huang AS, McIntosh K. A comparative study of virus isolation, polymerase chain reaction, and antigen detection in children of mothers infected with human immunodeficiency virus. J Pediatr 1990;116:372–376

MacDonald AB, Benach JL, Burgdorfer W. Stillbirth following maternal Lyme disease. N Y State J Med 1987;87:615–616

Markowitz LE, Steere AC, Benach JL, Slade JD, Broome CV. Lyme disease during pregnancy. JAMA 1986;255:3394–3396

Prober C, Sullender WM, Yasukawa LL, Au DS, Yeager AS, Arvin AM. Low risk of herpes simples virus infection in neonates exposed to the virus at the time of vaginal delivery to mothers with recurrent genital herpes simplex infection. N Engl J Med 1987;316:240–244

Rogers MF, Ou CY, Rayfield M, Thomas PA, Schoenbaum EE, Abrams E, et al. Use of the polymerase chain reaction for early detection of the proviral sequences of human immunodeficiency virus in infants born to seropositive mothers. N Engl J Med 1989;320:1649–1654

Schlesinger PA, Duray PH, Burke BA, Steere AC, Stillman MT. Maternal–fetal transmission of the Lyme disease spirochete, *Borrelia burgdorferi*. Ann Intern Med 1985;103:67–68

Scott GB, Hutto C, Makuch RW, Mastrucci MT, O'Connor T, Mitchell CD, et al. Survival in children with perinatally acquired human immunodeficiency virus type 1 infection. N Engl J Med 1989;321:1791–1796

Smith LG Jr, Pearlman M, Smith LG, Faro S. Lyme disease: a review with emphasis on the pregnant woman. Obstet Gynecol Surv 1991;46:125–130

Stagno S, Pass RF, Dworsky ME, Henderson RE, Moore EG, Walton PD, et al. Congenital cytomegalovirus infection: the relative importance of primary and recurrent maternal infection. N Engl J Med 1982;306:945–949

Williams CL, Benach JL, Curran AS, Spierling P, Medici F. Lyme disease during pregnancy: a cord blood serosurvey. N Y Acad Sci 1988;539:504

Williams CL, Strobino BA. Lyme disease transmission during pregnancy. Contemp Ob Gyn 1990;35(6):48–64

CHAPTER 6

INFECTION CONTROL

Infections are relatively uncommon in healthy mothers who deliver vaginally at term and in normal newborns. Women who have had prolonged rupture of membranes, with or without prolonged labor, are much more likely to develop infection, and sick or preterm neonates are infected relatively frequently.

Most infections in obstetric patients are caused by endogenous flora—microorganisms that are normally resident in the genital tract but generally cause no disease until labor, delivery, or the puerperium. Many of these infections can be prevented through meticulous surgical and patient care techniques and appropriate use of prophylactic antibiotics. Bacterial pathogens such as group B streptococci, *Listeria monocytogenes*, or *Chlamydia*, if acquired by neonates from their mothers in the intrapartum period, occasionally cause pneumonia or septicemia during the first hours or days of postnatal life. At present, these infections are difficult to predict or prevent, although they are known to occur more frequently after prolonged rupture of membranes or a complicated labor and delivery.

In contrast, most infections in neonates in intensive care units are caused by pathogens acquired from the hospital environment. The survival of more and more very-low-birth-weight infants; the emergence of chronic disease states, such as bronchopulmonary dysplasia; and the development of new invasive procedures provide additional opportunities for infectious problems to arise. Prevention of these infections requires a multifaceted approach, including meticulous patient care techniques, elimination of inappropriate antibiotic use to avoid further alteration of the balance of colonizing flora, and careful attention to all aspects of infection control.

Colonization in Neonates

Most neonates emerge from a sterile intrauterine environment. During and after birth, they are exposed to numerous microorganisms that colonize their skin, nasopharynx, and gastrointestinal tract, among other areas. Ill neonates who are subjected to multiple invasive procedures frequently have colonization at multiple sites with a variety of organisms, particularly gram-negative bacteria.

Severe infection in a full-term neonate is uncommon, but when it occurs it may be secondary to group B streptococci, *Escherichia coli* (particularly strains with K1 antigen), *L. monocytogenes*, *Citrobacter diversus*, *Salmonella*, *Chlamydia*, herpes simplex virus (HSV), or enteroviruses. These organisms can be transmitted to other neonates in the nursery on the hands of hospital personnel.

The skin of the newborn is a major initial site of bacterial colonization, particularly with *Staphylococcus aureus*; colonizing strains of this organism are most commonly transmitted within the nursery rather than from the mother. Any break in the integrity of the protective skin affords an opportunity for infection to develop. At birth, for example, a neonate has at least one open surgical wound (the umbilicus) that is highly susceptible to infection. A circumcision site is another area that is susceptible to infection.

Nursery Admission Policies

It is not necessary to restrict nursery admission to infants born under "sterile" conditions. Those born under "unsterile" conditions (eg, after prolonged rupture of membranes or to mothers with suspected or proved infection) or those transferred from a nursery at another hospital may be admitted to most nurseries if precautions are taken to prevent the transmission of colonizing or infecting organisms from one neonate to another. Similarly, neonates may be moved safely from one nursery area to another under normal circumstances. Categorizing neonates as "clean" or "dirty," based on whether they were born under sterile conditions, may lead to the assumption that the "clean" neonates do not harbor organisms that can cause disease, and this may result in inappropriate care. Each neonate should be approached as if he or she harbored colonies of unique flora that should not be transmitted to any other neonate. Personnel need to recognize the importance of proper infant care techniques in limiting the spread of organisms.

Neonatal Intensive Care

Neonates who require intensive care are highly susceptible to colonization. Because those neonates colonized with pathogenic organisms may have no overt signs of illness, special precautions may not be exercised in their care. Thus, physicians, nurses, respiratory therapy personnel, and other personnel who move from one neonate to another may carry these pathogenic organisms from neonates who have been colonized to those in the same nursery who have not yet been colonized. As a result, a high proportion of the neonates in a single nursery may be colonized or infected with the same strains of bacteria; respiratory tract and intestinal organisms are particularly common in such situations. To minimize the transmission of organisms, each individual working with these neonates and with the equipment used directly in their care should be meticulous when providing patient care. After taking care of one neonate, personnel should wash their hands before taking care of another neonate, and they should dispose of contaminated equipment or materials properly.

Surveillance for Nosocomial Infection

The infection control committee of each hospital should work with perinatal care personnel to establish workable definitions of nosocomial infection for surveillance purposes. For obstetric patients, a nosocomial infection can be broadly defined as one that is neither present nor incubating at the time the patient is admitted to the hospital. Most cases of endometritis or urinary tract infection that occur postpartum, therefore, are nosocomial, even though the causative organisms may be endogenous.

Nosocomial infection in newborns is more difficult to define. The broadest definition includes all infections that have an onset after birth, excluding only those known to have been transmitted transplacentally. Narrower definitions exclude those infections that develop within 24–72 hours of birth, because these, too, may have been caused by organisms acquired from the mother rather than from the hospital environment. The narrower, more specific definitions are probably more useful for general purposes. Definitions should include infections that become apparent within a certain period after a neonate's discharge. The definition selected should be applied consistently to allow uniform reporting and analysis of nosocomial infections.

Obstetric and nursery personnel should cooperate with hospital infection control personnel in conducting and reviewing the results of surveillance programs for nosocomial infections. This type of monitoring provides information about any unusual problems or clusters of infection, the risks associated with certain procedures or techniques, and the success of specific preventive measures. Generally, the surveillance program can be conducted most efficiently if it emphasizes the detection of infections in hospitalized patients, although most new mothers and their newborns are discharged after only a few days in the hospital.

Routine culturing of neonatal tissue for surveillance purposes is not recommended, but cultures of specimens from lesions or sites of infection can be helpful in identifying clusters of infection caused by a single strain of bacteria. As infections with organisms acquired within the nursery may not become apparent until after discharge of the newborns, it is especially important for pediatricians and others who care for the newborns to report confirmed or suspected postdischarge infections to nursery and hospital infection control personnel.

Patterns of infection are easier to recognize if the data include only those infections in which a specific site or pathogen can be identified. In neonates, however, it is frequently difficult to distinguish between the clinically insignificant presence of bacteria and disease at a site such as the lower respiratory tract. Usually, only clinically apparent infections should be recorded in the surveillance data; at times, especially during an outbreak of infection, it may be important to document organisms responsible for colonization of all neonates at certain sites. Clusters of infection that do not fit a standard definition may need to be individually investigated.

Both obstetric and nursery personnel are involved in providing perinatal care; therefore, close communication among these groups about infectious diseases is essential. In particular, nursery personnel should be notified in advance about the birth of a neonate who may have a congenital or perinatal infection, or about a mother who is known to be infected with, or to be a chronic carrier of, an organism (eg, *Salmonella*, hepatitis B virus [HBV], HSV, or human immune deficiency virus [HIV]). Conversely, obstetric personnel should be informed about problems in newborns that may be associated with labor and delivery or may have a bearing on maternal health.

Prevention and Control of Infections

Health Standards for Personnel

Obstetric and nursery personnel, as well as others who have significant contact with the newborn, should be free of transmissible infectious diseases. Each hospital should establish written policies and procedures for assessing the health of personnel assigned to the perinatal care services, restricting their contact with patients when necessary, maintaining their health records, and reporting any illness that they may have. These policies and procedures should address screening for tuberculosis and rubella. Routine culturing of specimens obtained from personnel is not useful, although selective culturing may be of value when a pattern of infection is suspected.

Personnel should be aware that even a mild transmissible infection may preclude contact with neonates. Ideally, individuals with a respiratory, cutaneous, mucocutaneous, hepatic, gastrointestinal, or other communicable infection should not have direct contact with neonates. Personnel who have exudative skin lesions or weeping dermatitis should refrain from all direct patient care and should not handle patient care equipment until the condition resolves. Personnel in contact with neonates should report personal infections or symptoms to their immediate supervisors and be medically examined before working directly with neonates. Decisions regarding the exclusion of staff members from obstetric and nursery areas should be made on an individual basis. Exclusion is appropriate for highly contagious conditions, even if the individual feels well enough to continue working. Employee health policies should be worded and applied in a way to ensure that personnel feel free to report infectious problems without fear of income loss.

Transmission of HSV from infected personnel to infants in newborn nurseries has been documented rarely. It is not known whether personnel who have labial HSV infection ("cold sores") or who are asymptomatic oral shedders of the virus can transmit the virus to infants, but the possibility seems extremely remote. The risk of compromising patient care by excluding personnel with "cold sores" when these personnel are essential for the operation of the nursery must be weighed against the potential risk of infecting newborn infants. Personnel with "cold sores" who have direct contact with infants should cover and avoid touching their lesions, and carefully observe hand-washing policies; furthermore, they should not kiss or nuzzle newborn infants or infants with eczema. Transmission of HSV infection from personnel with genital lesions is not likely, provided that hand-washing policies are carefully observed. Personnel with herpetic hand infections (herpetic whitlow) should not participate directly in the care of patients until the lesions have healed.

Personnel in neonatal units are likely to be exposed to patients excreting cytomegalovirus (CMV). There is no evidence that transfer to another area of the hospital or to a different group of patients decreases the risk, since many hospitalized patients asymptomatically excrete CMV. Acquisition of infection should be effectively prevented by simple measures, such as rigorous hand-washing after handling diapers or exposure to respiratory secretions and avoiding nuzzling and kissing infants. Because the majority of CMV infections are subclinical, previous infection and the current immune status of the exposed person are usually unknown. Women of childbearing age who work in neonatal units should be counseled about the relatively low risk of exposure should they become pregnant. Compliance with universal precautions, especially hand-washing, must be continually emphasized. Nurses should be given the option to be tested for immunity to CMV, but a routine program of serologic testing for obstetric or nursery hospital employees is not recommended.

It is desirable to recruit and maintain a regular group of nurses with specialized training in obstetric and neonatal nursing to work in these specialty areas. If nurses from other areas must work in the obstetric and neonatal care areas, or if nurses from the obstetric and neonatal care areas must work on other units of the hospital, specific policies should be established for this practice. Nursing personnel should not be moved indiscriminately between perinatal and nonperinatal areas.

Immunization

All hospital personnel, both men and women, who are susceptible to rubella should be immunized. Unless they are immunized, those working in the obstetric and nursery areas, including clinics, may contract the disease as a result of exposure to persons or neonates with rubella infection or may themselves transmit infection to pregnant women. Susceptible female personnel of childbearing age should be identified and offered immunization before they become pregnant or are exposed to infected patients. Vaccine should not be administered to pregnant women. There is no evidence that vaccine is teratogenic but, because the virus continues to shed, it is recommended that pregnancy be avoided for 3 months after vaccination. Should pregnancy occur, however, there is no evidence to support termination.

Influenza is likely to be serious or complicated in neonates, but they cannot be vaccinated against infection. Therefore, programs for immunization and chemoprophylaxis of adults who are in close contact with neonates may be an important means of protecting these infants from this disease. Annual immunization of nursery personnel against prevalent strains of influenza virus is strongly encouraged.

Precautions to Prevent Transmission of Blood-borne Pathogens

Medical history and examination do not reliably identify all patients infected with the blood-borne pathogens, such as HBV or HIV, that are of concern to health care personnel. For this reason, the Centers for Disease Control recommend that blood and body fluid precautions be used consistently for all patients. This approach, referred to as universal precautions, is particularly important when the risk of exposure to blood is high and the potential infectious status of the patient is not known.

The primary element of universal precautions is the use of appropriate barrier precautions by all health care personnel to prevent the exposure of their skin and mucous membranes to the blood or other body fluids of any patient. Gloves should be worn when it is necessary to have direct contact with blood and potentially infectious body fluids, mucous membranes, or nonintact skin of any patient; to handle items or surfaces soiled with blood or potentially infectious body fluids; and to perform venipuncture and other vascular access procedures. Hands should be washed immediately after the gloves are removed, and skin surfaces contaminated with blood or other potentially infectious material should be washed immediately and thoroughly.

Masks and protective eye wear or face shields should be worn during procedures that are likely to disperse droplets of blood or other body fluids, and gowns or aprons should be worn during procedures that are likely to generate splashes of these fluids (see "Dress Codes," this chapter).

All health care personnel should take precautions with needles, scalpels, and other sharp instruments in order to prevent injuries. Hospital infection control policies for handling and disposing of needles and other sharp objects should be clearly understood and followed by all personnel.

To avoid the need for emergency mouth-to-mouth resuscitation of patients, mouthpieces, endotracheal tubes, resuscitation bags and other ventilation devices, and suction equipment should be available for use in all areas where the need for resuscitation may arise.

Personnel caring for laboring and postpartum patients are frequently exposed to large amounts of blood and bloody body fluids; universal precautions must receive continual emphasis in these areas. In addition, perineal pads, sanitary napkins, and under-buttocks pads of all patients should be handled only with gloves and disposed of in a manner consistent with local infective waste statutes. Contaminated equipment should be appropriately bagged and sent for cleaning and disinfecting or sterilizing. Soiled linen should be placed in impermeable bags and appropriately labeled.

Hand-washing

Medical and hospital personnel must follow careful hand-washing techniques to minimize transmission of disease. Antiseptic preparations should be used for scrubbing before entering the nursery, before providing care for neonates highly susceptible to infection, before performing invasive procedures, and after providing care for infected neonates. For routine hand-washing within the nursery, soap and water may be sufficient.

The ideal antiseptic agent for hand-washing should kill pathogenic bacteria, be nonstaining and nonirritating to the skin, be nonsensitizing, and have persistent local action. It should also be easy to use. These requirements limit the number of useful preparations.

The antiseptics most useful for hand-washing in the nursery are chlorhexidine gluconate and iodophor preparations; both are useful against gram-negative and gram-positive organisms. Hexachlorophene-based preparations may be especially useful during nursery outbreaks of *S. aureus* infection, but they are not recommended for routine hand-washing. All the antiseptic compounds are occasionally sensitizing or irritating, and some personnel may need to use plain soap or mild detergents. Liquid soap dispensers and many hand-washing agents may become contaminated; disposable brushes or pads that contain an antiseptic hand-washing agent avoid this problem. Alcohol-containing foams kill bacteria satisfactorily when they are applied to clean hands, but they are not sufficient for cleaning physically soiled hands.

Before handling neonates for the first time on a shift, personnel should wash their hands and arms to a point above the elbow. A small amount of antiseptic preparation should be placed in the palm of the hand and the hands, wrists, forearms, and elbows washed thoroughly; all areas should be covered, including between the fingers and the lateral surfaces of the fifth fingers. Following this initial wash, the fingernails should be cleaned with a plastic or orangewood stick and the hands washed again (a soft brush or firm pad is optional). After the hands have been washed, they should be rinsed thoroughly and dried with paper towels.

A 10-second wash without a brush, but with soap and vigorous rubbing is required before and after handling each neonate and after touching objects or surfaces likely to be contaminated with virulent microorganisms or hospital pathogens (eg, the hair, face, or clothing of personnel; diapers; and equipment). This type of wash usually eliminates most organisms transiently colonizing the hands, although it may not be adequate if the hands are heavily contaminated. Routine, brief activities for the care of adult patients may not require hand-washing before each contact. Hand-washing facilities and materials must be easily accessible (see "Scrub Areas," Chapter 1).

Dress Codes

Each hospital should establish dress codes for regular and part-time personnel who enter the labor, delivery, and nursery areas. It is preferable for physicians, nursing personnel, and others who spend most of their working day in the labor or nursery areas to wear short-sleeved clothing, which may include scrub gowns or short-sleeved scrub suits or dresses provided and laundered by the hospital. Those who examine neonates should be sure that their clothing or unscrubbed portions of the body do not touch the neonates or any equipment. Fathers or other support person(s) attending births should be in scrub clothes. Sterile, long-sleeved gowns should be worn by all personnel who have direct contact with the sterile field during vaginal deliveries, surgical obstetric procedures, and surgical procedures in the nursery.

Some hospitals have approved more flexible dress codes for personnel who work in birthing rooms (eg, scrub suits without gowns or masks). Little information is available about the impact of these practices on the neonates, mothers, or personnel. Because of concern about potential infection of hospital personnel with blood-borne pathogens, such as HBV and HIV, the Centers for Disease Control recommend that all health care workers who perform or assist in deliveries wear gloves, gowns, surgical masks, and goggles during the procedure. Wearing aprons or gowns made of impervious material during cesarean delivery may provide additional protection. Gloves should be worn when handling the placenta or the neonate until blood and amniotic fluid have been removed from the neonate's skin. Hands should be washed immediately after gloves are removed or when skin surfaces are contaminated with blood.

In many nurseries where neonates are cared for in bassinets or open beds, physicians, nursing personnel, technicians who are not regularly assigned to the nursery, and visitors are required to wear short-sleeved gowns to cover their clothing. The need for this type of gowning as a routine infection control measure has not been confirmed, however.

If an infected or potentially infected neonate is to be handled outside the bassinet, a long-sleeved gown should be worn over the scrub suit or dress, gown, or other clothing and either discarded after use or maintained for use exclusively in the care of that neonate. If one gown is used for each neonate, the gowns should be changed every 8 hours.

Although caps, beard bags, and masks are not needed during routine activities in the labor and nursery areas, they are required during deliveries and may be beneficial during surgical procedures performed in the nursery, including umbilical vessel catheterization. Long hair should be restrained so that it does not touch the neonate or equipment during patient examination or treatments.

Masks have limitations; they are useful, but not usually essential, in preventing acquisition or dissemination of respiratory pathogens. High-efficiency, disposable masks should be used, but even these masks remain effective for only a few hours. Masks should be worn so that they cover both the nose and the mouth, and they should be discarded as soon as they are removed from the nose and mouth. Masks may not be effective on persons who have beards.

Sterile gloves should be used during deliveries and during all invasive procedures performed in either the obstetric (including birthing rooms) or the nursery area. Disposable, nonsterile gloves may be useful in the care of patients in isolation or in the performance of procedures that may result in heavy contamination of the hands. In such circumstances, the use of gloves may reduce the intensity of transient bacterial or viral colonization of the hands.

Personnel should remove rings, watches, and bracelets before washing their hands and entering the obstetric or nursery areas; they should not wear hand jewelry while on duty.

Suctioning

Personnel assisting in suctioning of the newborn should use mechanical devices. Equipment has been developed to allow wall suction to be used with valves that limit the amount of negative pressure generated and allow the individual to control when suctioning will occur. Direct wall suction should be avoided if possible, since most wall suction outlets have negative pressure levels that may be injurious.

Traditionally, mouth-suctioning devices such as the DeLee trap have been used to avoid getting aspirated material into the mouths of personnel. The use of mouth suctioning should be avoided. However, when mouth suction of the airway cannot be avoided, a trap should be placed in the line. (See also "Suctioning," Chapter 3.)

Obstetric Considerations

The trend toward relaxation of requirements regarding attire and conduct in family-centered perinatal programs and in-hospital birthing rooms has not been associated per se with a higher risk of infection in either mother or neonate. Current concerns over HIV infection, however, have resulted in stricter requirements as a safeguard to both patients and personnel. The delivery area should be considered a sterile area, especially when cesarean deliveries and tubal ligations are done in the same rooms in which vaginal deliveries are performed. Before surgery, the operative field should be prepared and draped. Shaving has been associated with a higher wound infection rate; when necessary, it should be done no earlier than 2 hours before surgery.

Monitoring

Intrauterine monitoring requires rupture of the amniotic membranes. To reduce the risk of infection in either the mother or the newborn, therefore, the catheter and leads should be carefully inserted by means of aseptic technique. Sterile equipment should be used for all fluid pathways in the pressure-monitoring system; the system should be closed, and extreme caution should be used to avoid contamination during procedures such as calibration.

Transducers for intravascular or intrauterine pressure monitoring have caused nosocomial infections for a variety of reasons. Contamination of equipment and subsequent infection in patients have resulted from suboptimal techniques in the assembly and use of equipment, from inadequate cleaning and sterilization of reusable equipment, and from the reuse of disposable transducer domes. To minimize the chance of inadvertent contamination of fluids and equipment, the components of the monitoring system should not be removed from sterile packages and set up until the system is actually needed. After use, all disposable equipment should be discarded and the transducer disinfected (if used with a disposable dome that isolates the head of the transducer from the fluid path) or cleaned and sterilized (if a reusable dome–transducer combination is used). Disposable pressure assemblies are now available and, although more expensive, may have a distinct advantage in decreasing the risk of infection.

Genital Infection (Endometritis)

Endometritis occurs after 1–3% of vaginal deliveries and complicates 10–50% of cesarean deliveries. Furthermore, genital infections are frequently more severe after cesarean delivery than after vaginal delivery. Risk factors for infection include prolonged labor or rupture of membranes, lower socioeconomic status, anemia, and trauma. The results of most studies indicate that internal fetal monitoring does not directly increase infection rates in the mother. Endometritis, which usually appears within the first few days after delivery, is characterized by fever, malaise, tachycardia, abdominal pain, or foul lochia. There may be no localizing signs early in the course of infection.

Management. The condition of febrile postpartum patients (temperature ≥102°F) should be evaluated by means of a pertinent history, complete physical examination, blood count, and urine cultures. Blood cultures may be indicated with suspected serious infections. Bacteria most likely to cause infection are the gram-negative enteric aerobes (especially *E. coli*), selected aerobic streptococci (group B α-hemolytic streptococci, and the enterococci), gram-negative anaerobic rods (especially *Bacteroides bivius*), and anaerobic cocci (*Peptococcus* and *Peptostreptococcus*). Infections are often mixed. Isolation procedures are appropriate for infrequent cases caused by group A streptococci (see "Infected Postpartum Patients," this chapter); wound precautions are appropriate for women with draining abdominal incisions.

Patients usually respond promptly to antibiotic therapy, but persistent fever, retained infected placenta, septic pelvic thrombophlebitis, or pelvic abscess are occasional complications.

Prophylaxis Against Postcesarean Endometritis. Well-designed studies have demonstrated that short-course prophylaxis significantly decreases endometritis after nonelective cesarean delivery (ie, cesarean delivery after rupture of membranes or labor of any duration). Administration of intravenous antibiotic immediately after cord clamping or by uterine irrigation following placental removal has been demonstrated to be as effective as beginning it before surgery. For procedures lasting less than 2 hours, a single dose is as effective as a longer course. If massive intraoperative blood loss occurs, a second dose may be indicated.

The choice of antibiotic for cesarean delivery prophylaxis varies. Most studies have found ampicillin or a first-generation cephalosporin to be as effective as other broader spectrum agents.

Neonatal Considerations

Invasive Procedures on Neonates

Percutaneous placement of peripheral arterial or venous cannulas is associated with a lower risk of infection than is placement by surgical cutdown. They should be removed promptly if clinical signs suggest infection. A safe maximal duration of cannulation for intravascular catheters has not been established; a careful daily assessment of risks versus benefits should be made for each neonate. Intravascular catheters should not be used or left in place unless clearly indicated for medical management of the neonate. Each unit should have a written policy on the management of these catheters.

Arterial cannulas represent an ideal pressure-monitoring device in a closed system, but they frequently are also used for obtaining blood samples. These samples should be obtained aseptically with precautions to avoid contamination of the system (eg, from ice used to chill syringes before obtaining the blood sample). Because some species of bacteria flourish in dextrose solutions at room temperature, this type of solution should not be used in pressure-monitoring systems unless absolutely necessary.

Total parenteral nutrition generally is a safe technique but it has been associated with infection, including septicemia and fungemia. A cooperative team approach that involves pharmacists, nurses, and physicians is strongly recommended, as such an approach reduces the incidence of infections and other complications. Meticulous attention should be paid to aseptic insertion and maintenance of the cannula and to aseptic techniques of fluid administration. All parenteral nutrition fluids should be mixed in a central pharmacy, preferably in a laminar flow hood. Because lipid emulsions are especially susceptible to contamination with a wide variety of bacteria and fungi that can proliferate to high concentrations within hours, particular caution must be taken in the storage and administration of these emulsions. Unit-dose amounts may be delivered from the pharmacy; if bottles of emulsion are kept in the nursery refrigerator, care should be taken to prevent contamination. Opened bottles must be discarded no later than 24 hours after the seal has been broken.

Intravascular Flush Solutions

The hospital pharmacy should establish a system to ensure a satisfactory and safe means of providing sterile, unpreserved fluids to the nursery areas. When administered to neonates, solutions with benzyl alcohol may lead to severe metabolic acidosis, encephalopathy, and even death. If the fluid administered is to contain heparin, it should be added to the fluid in the hospital pharmacy whenever possible. Flush solutions should be kept at room temperature no longer than 8 hours before being used or discarded.

Antibiotics

The efficacy of antibiotics used for prophylaxis in newborns has not been documented, and such use should be strongly discouraged. Topical antibiotics should be used only for very specific indications and only on the order of a physician. The indiscriminate and inappropriate use of either systemic or topical antibiotics may alter the established flora of the neonate and result in the emergence of resistant strains of bacteria, making subsequent therapy for clinical infections more difficult and dangerous. In addition, systemic prophylactic therapy may alter the clinical expression of infection, making diagnosis more difficult and delaying appropriate antimicrobial therapy.

The relative frequencies of documented infection with different bacteria in neonates, along with patterns of antimicrobial susceptibility, should be monitored by the infection control committee. The most innocuous and specific antibiotic regimens should be selected after analysis of these data. For example, if kanamycin-resistant, gram-negative bacteria only rarely cause infections during the first week of postnatal life, but cause infections more frequently in older infants, kanamycin can be used selectively in the younger group.

Skin Care of the Newborn

Effects on the skin should be considered in selecting skin care techniques. Some agents are absorbed and may be toxic; others change skin flora and may give rise to infectious problems.

Cleansing should be delayed until the neonate's temperature has stabilized. Whole-body bathing of the infant may not be necessary. Localized skin care or techniques that minimize exposure to water may reduce the neonate's heat loss. Sterile cotton sponges (not gauze) soaked with warm water may be used to remove blood and meconium from the neonate's face, head, and body. Alternatively, a mild, nonmedicated soap, preferably in a single-use container or in a small bar reserved for a single neonate, can be used and rinsed with water. Careful drying of the neonate's skin and removal of blood after birth may minimize the risk of infection with potentially contaminating microorganisms, such as HBV, HSV, and HIV. If the neonate's skin is not grossly soiled, it may not require much cleansing. The vernix caseosa may have a protective function, although some believe it does not; there is no evidence to indicate that it is harmful, however.

For the remainder of the neonate's stay in the hospital nursery, the buttocks and perianal regions should be cleansed with fresh water and cotton, with a mild soap and water at diaper changes, or as often as required.

Various antiseptic compounds for skin care have been studied to determine their safety and effectiveness in preventing colonization and infection in neonates. Hexachlorophene, while relatively effective against gram-positive bacteria, particularly *S. aureus*, should not be used routinely for bathing neonates because it may be absorbed through intact skin and is potentially neurotoxic for neonates. Although they are good antiseptics, iodophors have not been proved both safe and effective for routine skin care to prevent colonization and disease in newborns. Chlorhexidine gluconate, a compound that is poorly absorbed through intact skin, is useful for bathing or localized skin care.

No single method of cord care has proved superior in preventing colonization and disease. Current methods include the local application of antimicrobial agents, such as bacitracin, or of triple dye. The skin absorption and toxicity of the triple dye agents in newborns have not been carefully studied. Alcohol hastens the drying of the cord, but, although frequently used as an antiseptic, is probably not effective in preventing cord colonization and omphalitis.

Ideally, agents used on the newborn's skin should be dispensed in single-use containers, or each patient should have a personal dispenser.

Immunization of Premature Neonates and Long-term Nursery Residents

The following immunization guidelines for preterm infants (whether hospitalized or not) are based on the premise that premature infants do not have significant antibody that will interfere with immunization and that most of these infants have the ability to produce immunoglobulins M and G when stimulated with a variety of antigens:

- All neonatal intensive care nurseries should implement a policy for immunization of premature infants.

- Preterm infants can be given diphtheria, tetanus, and pertussis (DTP) vaccine and oral polio vaccine (OPV) at the appropriate chronologic age (ie, 2 months). Half-dose DTP should not be used.

- If the infant remains in the hospital, only DTP should be given to avoid cross-infection with OPV in the nursery; the OPV series can be initiated on discharge. DTP should be given at least 48 hours prior to discharge to permit observation of side reactions. Alternatively, inactivated polio vaccine can be considered for infants with long lengths of stay.

- If the infant leaves the hospital at 2 months of age, both DTP and OPV can be given on discharge.

- Contraindications for DTP administration in premature infants are the same as those for full-term infants.

- Although the response of premature infants to Haemophilus influenzae type B vaccine is currently unknown, the first H. influenzae type B immunization should be given at 2 months of chronologic age.

Isolation

The current system of patient isolation recommended for most hospitals in the United States is designed around seven basic categories:

1. Strict isolation
2. Respiratory isolation
3. Contact isolation
4. Drainage/secretion precautions
5. Enteric precautions
6. Blood/body fluid precautions
7. Tuberculosis isolation

Detailed descriptions of the isolation categories and requirements are provided in *Guidelines for Isolation Precautions in Hospitals.* The isolation categories were not designed for the special needs of neonates and nurseries, however, so specific procedures used within each category may need modification for neonates.

Infected Postpartum Patients

Patients with group A streptococcal puerperal endometritis should be managed with contact isolation until 24 hours after the initiation of adequate antimicrobial therapy; a private room is desirable, particularly if patient hygiene is poor. A gown and gloves should be used for direct contact with the infected area or drainage. Patients with abscesses or draining infections of the perineum or of abdominal wounds should be managed with drainage/secretion precautions, or contact isolation; if a dressing does not adequately contain the wound discharge, a private room may be desirable.

Control measures needed in the care of febrile puerperal patients will depend on the likely clinical diagnosis. Careful attention to aseptic patient care techniques, universal precautions, and meticulous hand-washing after contact with patients, especially after direct contact with infected areas, are essential.

Postpartum patients with communicable diseases that are not unique to obstetric patients should be managed with appropriate precautions or isolation. If there is a significant risk that such a disease will be transmitted to other patients or if the necessary procedures cannot be performed adequately on the obstetric unit, such patients should be transferred to another nursing unit that can provide proper care.

Contact of Neonates with Their Infected Mothers

Most maternal genital infections, with the exception of group A streptococcal disease, are caused by endogenous microorganisms that ascend into the uterus from the lower genital tract; postnatal spread of infection from this site to neonates is rare. Consequently, a febrile postpartum woman without a specifically identified site of infection usually may be allowed to handle and feed her newborn if she 1) is feeling well enough; 2) washes her hands thoroughly, under supervision; and 3) wears a clean hospital cover gown to prevent contact of the neonate with contaminated items, such as bedclothes, pads, and linen. A woman with a communicable disease that is likely to be transmitted to her newborn should be separated from the newborn until the infection is no longer communicable.

A mother with a respiratory tract infection should be fully informed that such infections are easily transmitted on hands or by fomites, and she should be instructed in careful hand-washing techniques and appropriate handling of tissues or other items contaminated with infectious secretions. It may be wise for her to use a surgical mask when she is with her newborn to reduce the chance of droplet spread of infection.

Breast-feeding is usually possible even if the mother has an overt infection or if she is receiving antibiotics. Although antibiotics are secreted in breast milk in small amounts, this is usually not a contraindication to the continuation of breast-feeding (see Chapter 7).

Cohorts

In large nurseries, cohorts of neonates may be established to minimize transmission of microorganisms or infectious diseases among different groups of neonates. A cohort usually consists of well neonates born during the same 24- or 48-hour period; these neonates are kept in a single nursery room and, ideally, are cared for by a single group of personnel who do not care for any other cohort during a given shift. After the neonates in a cohort have been discharged, the room should be thoroughly cleaned and prepared to accept the next cohort.

The use of cohorts is not usually practical for small hospitals or for those facilities with intensive care and graded care units. Even in these facilities, however, this approach can be useful in efforts to control epidemics or in the management of a group of neonates colonized or infected with a specific microbial strain. Although separate rooms for these cohorts are ideal, they are not mandatory if there is a means to demarcate cohort lines within a single large room and if personnel assigned to a cohort provide care only for neonates in that cohort.

During an epidemic, neonates with overt infection and those who are colonized should be identified rapidly and placed in cohorts. If rapid identification of these neonates is not possible, separate cohorts should be established for neonates with disease, those who have been exposed, those who have not been exposed, and those who are newly admitted. The success of cohort programs depends largely on the willingness and ability of nursery and ancillary personnel to adhere strictly to the cohort system and to follow established practices.

Neonates with Suspected or Proved Infections

The housing of an infected neonate depends on the overall condition of the neonate and the type of care required, the available space and facilities, the nurse/patient ratio, and the size and type of the neonatal care service. Other factors to be considered include the type of infection (ie, specific viral or bacterial pathogen), the clinical manifestations, the infection's source and the possible modes of its transmission, and the number of colonized or infected neonates.

In many instances (notable exceptions are neonatal varicella and HSV infections), isolation rooms are unnecessary for infected neonates if 1) sufficient nursing and medical staff are on duty to provide comprehensive care, 2) there is sufficient space for a 4–6-ft aisle or area between neonatal stations, 3) two or more sinks for hand-washing are available in each nursery room or area, and 4) continuing instruction is provided about the ways in which infections spread. If these criteria are not met, an isolation room with separate scrub facilities is necessary.

It has often been assumed that forced-air incubators provide adequate isolation for infected neonates. While these incubators filter incoming air, they do not filter the air that is discharged into the nursery. They are satisfactory, therefore, for limited protective isolation of neonates; they should not be relied on to prevent transmission of microorganisms from infected neonates to others, however, because the surfaces of incubators are readily contaminated with the microorganisms that have infected or colonized the neonates.

Gastroenteritis or Draining Lesions. It is easiest to isolate neonates with gastroenteritis (diarrhea), draining lesions (eg, caused by *S. aureus*), or purulent conjunctivitis by placing them in a separate or isolation room. They may be treated in the general newborn, intermediate, or intensive care areas, provided that these areas are adequately staffed and have sufficient space and equipment to allow isolation and proper care. The most important factor in preventing the spread of infection is the presence of sufficient nursing personnel. If more than one neonate is infected, a cohort approach should be taken.

Enteric precautions or drainage/secretion precautions should be observed. All personnel should use a gown and disposable gloves when providing direct patient care. Contaminated items should be discarded properly. The environment may be heavily contaminated with the infecting microorganism, and transmission of these organisms to other neonates often occurs on the hands of personnel.

Congenital Infections. For neonates with congenital infections the Centers for Disease Control recommend the following isolation precautions:

- Congenital rubella: contact isolation (mask, gown, gloves, private room)
- Congenital syphilis: both drainage/secretion precautions and blood/body fluid precautions
- Cytomegalovirus infection: urine and respiratory secretion precautions
- Toxoplasmosis: no isolation necessary
- Herpes simplex: contact isolation for clinically infected neonates or those delivered either vaginally or by cesarean birth to women with active genital herpes simplex infections

Viral Infections. Many viruses, such as respiratory syncytial virus, coxsackieviruses, or echoviruses, spread rapidly among neonates and personnel in a nursery. Such viral infections can be serious in neonates, sometimes resulting in death. As neonates may shed selected viruses after their clinical illness has been resolved, they become reservoirs of infection. It is believed that the viruses are transmitted predominantly by direct or indirect contact with the contaminated hands of personnel or with contaminated environmental surfaces or fomites. Contact isolation may be required to prevent this type of spread, but specific requirements vary with the infecting virus. For example, respiratory syncytial virus is shed primarily from the respiratory tract, while coxsackieviruses or echoviruses can be shed from the throat or in the stool.

Neonates are usually ineffective disseminators of infectious bacterial or viral aerosols. Neonates with confirmed or possible infections caused by a viral agent that could be transmitted by the airborne route should be separated from other neonates 1) by transfer from the nursery area, 2) by rooming-in with the mother, or 3) by enclosure of all other neonates in the area in incubators (ie, reverse isolation).

Management of Nursery Outbreaks of Disease

Because many infections become apparent only after neonates leave the hospital, each hospital should establish a procedure to be used during a suspected or confirmed epidemic for disease surveillance of recently discharged neonates. Procedures for control of nursery epidemics depend on the microorganism responsible for the outbreak, the reservoir of infection, and the mode of transmission. An epidemiologic investigation should be undertaken to identify these factors. The hospital infection control committee and the proper health authorities should be notified promptly about all suspected or confirmed epidemics.

During epidemics, a comprehensive program of infection control is required. If a problem is suspected, the first step is to evaluate it promptly and carefully. The result of this initial assessment determines the need for further epidemiologic studies to define the source and means of transmission of the infections, as well as the type of specific control measures that are required. Even if an intensive investigation is not indicated, the results of the control measures should be evaluated to ensure that they have been effective and the problem has been resolved.

Staphylococcus aureus

Colonization of newborns by *S. aureus* is relatively common, but disease is usually sporadic; the frequency of disease is dependent on multiple factors, including the virulence of the colonizing strain. Although the prevalence of *S. aureus* colonization of neonates fluctuates and may at times be more than 50%, nurseries with good infection control practices are often able to restrict neonate colonization rates to 20% or less. Disease may occur with any prevalence of colonization in the nursery, however. The incubation period for staphylococcal lesions is highly variable. Most frequently, disease caused by infection with *S. aureus* occurs in neonates during the second week of postnatal life, after the neonates have been discharged from the nursery. Infections detected in neonates before discharge from the nursery, therefore, may represent only a small fraction of the total.

Generally, *S. aureus* is transmitted to neonates on the inadequately washed hands of personnel; colonized and infected neonates serve as the reservoir. Rarely, a personnel disseminator, with or without staphylococcal lesions, is responsible for a cluster of infection. Most colonized personnel do not disseminate their organisms, however, and the colonization is insignificant epidemiologically. The carriers require no special treatment, and routine culturing of specimens from hospital personnel is not recommended. Fomites are not usually implicated in the transmission of *S. aureus* infections.

A presumptive epidemic in a nursery may be defined as the occurrence of cutaneous infection in two or more neonates simultaneously (or within a short period of time), the development of a breast abscess in a mother, or a deep infection in a neonate. Another rough guideline is that no more than three or four full-term neonates per 1,000 live births should develop *S. aureus* infection while in the nursery. If an epidemic or infection with methicillin-resistant *S. aureus* is suspected, the following approaches should be considered:

- Careful hand-washing by personnel is of paramount importance.

- Infants with definite or suspected staphylococcal disease should be placed in strict isolation.

- Basic patient care techniques should be reemphasized and cohorts instituted for infected, colonized, and newly admitted neonates. All neonates in a room should be discharged and the room carefully cleaned before other neonates are admitted to that room. A strictly enforced cohort system for both neonates and personnel virtually eliminates contact between infected and uninfected neonates, interrupting disease transmission.

- The extent of disease in neonates recently discharged from the hospital should be determined, either by a survey of the physicians or health care providers who take care of most neonates born in the hospital or by a survey of the parents of these neonates. Health departments or nursing associations may provide assistance with the survey.

- Specimens obtained from the umbilical stump of infants and the anterior nares of personnel should be cultured to determine the prevalence of colonization and to identify the staphylococcal strains involved in the outbreak for antibiotic sensitivity testing and phage typing. Occasionally, it is necessary to identify personnel colonized with a strain that has been implicated in epidemic disease in a closed population and to remove these carriers from areas of patient contact. These personnel should be treated with topical intranasal antibiotics; sometimes, orally administered antibiotics are also necessary. The goal of therapy is to eliminate carriage of an epidemiologically virulent strain, which may be extremely difficult.

- During periods of epidemic disease, full-term infants may be bathed, in the diaper area only, with hexachlorophene (3%) as soon after birth as possible and daily until they are discharged. The hexachlorophene should be thoroughly washed off after bathing is completed and should not be used for routine bathing. Hexachlorophene should be used only for full-term infants.

- Application of triple dye or bacitracin ointment to the umbilical stump of all infants twice daily throughout the nursery stay may be helpful.

- In unusual circumstances, it may be necessary to give oral antistaphylococcal agents to all infants and personnel who are carriers.

- Persons involved in hospital outbreaks of staphylococcal disease should be observed and warned of the possibility of delayed disease and the spread to family members.

- Surveillance in the nursery should be continued for several weeks after the epidemic has apparently terminated. Observation for disease in neonates (both in the nursery and at home for several weeks after discharge) is the most reliable index. Weekly cultures of specimens from the umbilical cord and nares of neonates in the nursery and of specimens from the nares of personnel may be valuable for a short time, but long periods of serial surveillance of neonates and personnel are not practical. Monitoring of neonates for *S. aureus* is probably the best method for determining the need for prevalence surveys in neonates or personnel.

Infectious Diarrhea: Escherichia coli

Measures for the management of a nursery epidemic of diarrheal disease caused by *E. coli* are also appropriate for the management of diarrheal disease caused by other bacterial (eg, *Salmonella*) or viral pathogens. The reservoir of infection is usually the intestinal tract of ill or colonized neonates, and infection is usually transmitted from neonate to neonate on the inadequately washed hands of personnel. Occasionally, other sources, such as extrinsically contaminated formula, may be found.

Epidemic enteric disease may be caused by 1) strains of enterotoxin-producing *E. coli* that may or may not be agglutinated by commercial antisera or 2) specific enteropathogenic *E. coli* that do not usually produce known enterotoxins. Strains of *E. coli* can be identified by their colony characteristics and antimicrobial susceptibility patterns; when a single strain is predominant or pure in cultures from ill neonates, when the strain is isolated from ill neonates much more often than from those who remain well, and when there is no other obvious pathogen such as *Shigella* or *Salmonella*, that strain is likely to be the epidemic strain. It should be serotyped and tested for enterotoxin production if this can be done quickly and reliably by available laboratories.

Because asymptomatic carriage of an identifiable pathogen may perpetuate an outbreak, a rectal specimen for culture should be obtained from neonates in proximity to the index case or to other symptomatic neonates.

Diseased and colonized neonates should be placed into strict cohorts and segregated from the other neonates; personnel providing care for the culture-positive neonates should not provide care for neonates who have not been infected or colonized. If possible, it is helpful to reduce the number of neonates in the nursery. If multiple cases occur, the nursery room should be closed to admissions and not reopened until all neonates in the room have been discharged and the room has been cleaned. Newborns should be discharged home, not transferred to other nurseries. In some outbreaks, it may be necessary to close the entire nursery to all new admissions and to make other arrangements for newborns.

Appropriate antibiotics should be administered to all neonates excreting the epidemic strain. If serotype information is not available to identify the epidemic strain, all symptomatic neonates, as well as those in the same room or cohort, should be treated. Antibiotic selection should be based on susceptibility tests. Colistin (10–15 mg/kg per day) or neomycin (100 mg/kg per day), administered orally in three or four doses for 5 days, may be useful. Although treatment of this duration may be adequate, neonates who must remain in the nursery should be retreated if they continue to carry the pathogenic strain (as determined by fluorescent antibody study or culture of three consecutive specimens obtained after completion of antibiotic therapy). During an outbreak, prophylactic administration of colistin or neomycin to all neonates may be appropriate, although efficacy may be variable.

Personnel who are carriers of the epidemic organism have been implicated only rarely as the source of an epidemic, but they should be identified by culture of stool specimens. Carrier–disseminators should be removed from the nursery until they have been treated and are culture negative.

Antiseptic and aseptic techniques should be reviewed and strictly observed. Particular emphasis should be placed on hand-washing by personnel before and after each contact with each neonate. Body fluid isolation should be practiced with all neonates whether or not they are infected. Requiring personnel to wear gowns and gloves when caring for infected or colonized neonates and to wash their hands after handling infected neonates and contaminated materials may reduce the degree of contamination of hands and clothing by the infecting pathogen.

Although *E. coli* is seldom transmitted from neonate to neonate by means of contaminated fomites, nursery practices should be evaluated; equipment that may be contaminated, especially solutions or articles that would have contact with the gastrointestinal tract of neonates, may need to be cultured. After all infected or colonized neonates have been discharged, the nursery, including the equipment, should be thoroughly cleaned and disinfected.

Neonates recently discharged should be surveyed. All symptomatic neonates should be examined, specimens obtained for culture, and treatment provided. Surveillance by periodic examination of cultures from neonates, personnel, and other sources of contamination should be continued for a short period after the outbreak has been controlled. If the pathogen is not recovered from cultures, surveillance can be ended.

Klebsiella and Other Gram-Negative Bacteria

Gram-negative bacteria, especially *Klebsiella pneumoniae*, frequently cause infections in nurseries, particularly in intensive care nurseries. Strains of these bacteria that are resistant to various antibiotics, including gentamicin, kanamycin, and chloramphenicol, are becoming increasingly common. Thus, these organisms may be virulent, invasive, and unusually difficult to eradicate.

The physician in charge of the nursery should be aware of all illness in the neonates and the nature of infections in personnel so that clusters of infections are recognized and appropriately investigated. Because nursery-acquired infections may become evident only several weeks to months after discharge, this physician should be notified by other physicians in the community of serious infections in infants who have recently been discharged from the nursery.

Several cases of infection occurring in infants in physical proximity or caused by an unusual pathogen may indicate an epidemic, in which case epidemiologic or bacteriologic surveys may be necessary to identify the source. When these surveys confirm an epidemic, infection-control procedures should be instituted promptly. Although clinical infection with *Klebsiella* and other gram-negative bacteria may occur at various sites, the intestinal tract is the most frequent site of colonization; therefore, stool cultures (and perhaps cultures of specimens from other sites) should be obtained from all neonates in the nursery to identify rapidly those who are colonized. Selective media containing antibiotics may be used to simplify isolation of the specific pathogen.

The infected neonates should be segregated and managed with appropriate isolation precautions (eg, contact isolation or enteric precautions). Neonate isolation techniques should include the use of disposable diapers and gloves. A strict cohort system should be established immediately. Personnel providing care for infected or colonized neonates should not provide care for uninfected neonates, as transmission appears to occur despite careful hand-washing. The pattern of antibiotic use in the nursery may have to be altered periodically to avoid bacterial resistance.

Necrotizing Enterocolitis

The etiology and pathophysiology of necrotizing enterocolitis are poorly understood. Cases often occur in clusters, and several investigators have noted that neonates whose bowel has been colonized by specific strains of bacteria are more likely to develop necrotizing enterocolitis than are neonates colonized by different strains. These data suggest that it may be prudent to manage neonates with suspected or confirmed necrotizing enterocolitis with enteric precautions, including the use of gown and gloves when working directly with the neonate or articles likely to be contaminated with feces. A cluster of cases may require the establishment of a strict cohort of neonates colonized with a common bacterial strain. A cohort of personnel should also be established to care for the affected neonates.

Administration of prophylactic oral or systemic antibiotics in an effort to prevent necrotizing enterocolitis in neonates has not been successful and is likely to result in the emergence of resistant bacteria.

Group A Streptococci

Epidemics of infection with strains of group A streptococci are uncommon at present. If this problem should arise, the following steps are recommended:

- Determine the extent of the epidemic by culturing any lesions and the umbilical stumps of all neonates in the nursery.

- Institute a cohort system. The nursery need not be closed to new admissions.

- Employ the various approaches that have been used to control epidemics, including isolation and treatment of all culture-positive neonates (cohort isolation is satisfactory), fomite control, and careful hand-washing. A complete epidemiologic investigation with isolation or treatment of carriers is essential to control. Use body-substance isolation techniques for all neonates. In order to reduce the number of neonates in the nursery who may serve as a reservoir for infection, cohort those neonates who are infected, colonized, or exposed.

- Provide prophylaxis for all neonates with penicillin G benzathine (50,000 U/kg intramuscularly); treat neonates with disease caused by group A streptococci with penicillin G (50,000–100,000 U/kg per day intravenously in two or three divided doses) for 10 days.

- Conduct a telephone survey of the parents or pediatricians of recently discharged, exposed neonates to determine whether any neonate is ill (although most neonates carrying group A streptococci will be free of disease or will have only a mild omphalitis). Examine symptomatic neonates and obtain specimens for culture; institute antibiotic treatment, if appropriate.

- Obtain culture specimens from the nose, throat, and any cutaneous lesion of all nursery personnel. Anal carriage of group A streptococci has been implicated as the cause of epidemics of surgical wound infections; to avoid the need for anal cultures from all nursery personnel, epidemiologic techniques should be used in an effort to identify those few personnel most likely to be disseminating infection. Personnel with positive cultures should be removed from the nursery and treated until cultures are negative.

- Continue surveillance in the nursery for several weeks after the epidemic has ended. Obtain specimens for culture from neonates just before they are discharged. If the problem persists, weekly nose and throat cultures of nursery personnel may be indicated.

Environmental Control

The physician in charge and the nursing supervisor of the obstetric and nursery areas should work with the infection control officer and other groups as appropriate (eg, representatives of the respiratory therapy service, central supply, and housekeeping) to establish an environmental control program for the labor, delivery, and nursery areas. This program should include specific procedures in a written policy manual for cleaning and disinfection or sterilization of patient care areas, equipment, and supplies. Consultation for specific details and problems is essential. Nursing supervisors should ensure that these procedures are carried out correctly.

Methods of Sterilization and Disinfection

All medical and hospital personnel should understand the difference between sterilization and disinfection. Sterilization is the destruction of all microorganisms, including spores; disinfection is simply a reduction in the number of contaminating microorganisms. High-level disinfection is the elimination or destruction of all microorganisms, except spores. Cleaning is the physical removal of organic material or soil, including microorganisms, from objects.

Equipment that enters normally sterile tissue or the vascular system should be sterile. For neonates, equipment that comes into contact with mucous membranes or that has prolonged or intimate contact with skin should also be sterile. Much of the equipment required in perinatal care areas can be used safely if it is satisfactorily cleaned and disinfected, however; clean, dry surfaces do not support the growth of microorganisms.

It is sometimes necessary to decontaminate equipment before it is cleaned and sterilized or disinfected in order to allow processing without the risk of exposure of personnel to hazardous microbes. The equipment must be cleaned thoroughly to remove all blood, tissue, secretions, food, and other residue. Without thorough cleaning, no method of sterilization or disinfection can be effective. Furthermore, some chemical disinfectants are inactivated by organic materials.

Sterilization

Methods of sterilization include steam autoclaving, dry heat, and gaseous (ethylene oxide) or liquid chemical (eg, 2% glutaraldehyde) techniques. The preferred method of sterilization is steam autoclaving, because this is the least expensive method and provides the greatest margin of safety. Some equipment may be damaged by steam, however, and must be sterilized by another method.

Equipment made of material that absorbs ethylene oxide usually requires 8–12 hours of aeration after sterilization with ethylene oxide before it can be used again. Ethylene oxide sterilization of supplies or equipment should be preceded by a comprehensive review of authoritative data on the aeration time required for each material to be processed and the extent to which toxicity standards have been established. An ethylene oxide sterilization plan requires the presence of sufficient backup equipment to allow time for aeration.

Equipment that cannot be sterilized with steam or ethylene oxide may be satisfactorily sterilized after cleaning by immersion for 10 hours in 2% glutaraldehyde or other acceptable liquid sporicide; this should be followed by three rinses with sterile water (or tap water with at least 10 mg of hypochlorite per liter), thorough drying, and packaging in sterile wrappers.

High-Level Disinfection

Equipment that does not need to be sterilized may be subjected to high-level disinfection. Both hot-water pasteurization and chemical disinfection are satisfactory. Pasteurization of equipment requires immersing it in water at 80–85°C (176–185°F) for 15 minutes or 75°C (167°F) for 30 minutes. After air drying (preferably in a cabinet with heated, filtered air), disinfected items should be aseptically wrapped and stored until needed. Although spores are not eradicated by this method, bacterial and viral decontamination is adequate. The original reports of the equipment manufacturer should be consulted for a list of any parts or materials that may be warped or damaged at these temperatures.

The choice of liquid chemicals for high-level disinfection depends on the type of equipment to be disinfected. In many instances, immersion of the equipment for 30 minutes in 2% glutaraldehyde or an environmental iodophor solution (500 ppm available iodine), followed by three rinses with sterile water (or tap water with at least 10 mg of hypochlorite per liter) and thorough drying, is satisfactory.

Cleaning and Disinfecting Noncritical Surfaces

Selection of Disinfectants

Although numerous disinfectants are available, no single agent or preparation is ideal for all purposes. Consideration should be given to the agent and its special use as well as to the types of organisms likely to be contaminating the object that is to be disinfected. Special attention should be given to the recommended concentration of each disinfectant and its time of exposure. Unnecessary exposure of neonates to disinfectants should be avoided, and strict adherence to manufacturers' recommendations is essential.

Hexachlorophene preparations are not disinfectants and should not be used on equipment or environmental surfaces. Iodophors, chlorine compounds, phenolic compounds, and glutaraldehyde are satisfactory disinfectants. Only iodophor or quaternary disinfectant detergent products should be used that are registered by the U.S. Environmental Protection Agency and recommended by the manufacturer for nursery surfaces with which neonates have contact. Phenolic compounds, especially if used in inappropriate concentrations or on surfaces with which neonates have direct contact, have been associated with hyperbilirubinemia. Information about specific label claims of commercial germicides can be obtained by writing to the Disinfectants Branch, Office of Pesticides, Environmental Protection Agency, 401 M Street, SW, Washington, DC 20460.

General Housekeeping

The following order of cleaning is recommended:

1. Patient areas
2. Accessory areas
3. Adjacent halls

It is not known whether floor bacteria are a source of nosocomial infection, but regular cleaning prevents the accumulation of pathogenic bacteria. Disinfectant–detergents have been shown to be more effective than soap and water alone in cleaning floors, although hospital floors are rapidly recontaminated after disinfection. Available disinfectant–detergents may differ in effectiveness.

In the cleaning procedure, dust should not be dispersed into the air. Removal of dust by a dry vacuum machine, followed by wet vacuuming, is effective in cleaning and disinfecting hospital floors. Once dust has been removed, scrubbing with a mop and a disinfectant–detergent solution should be sufficient. Mop heads should be machine-laundered and thoroughly dried daily.

Standard types of portable vacuum cleaners should not be used in nurseries or delivery areas because particulate matter and microbial contamination in the room may be disturbed and distributed by the exhaust jet. Vacuum cleaners that discharge outside the patient care area (ie, central vacuum cleaning systems or portable vacuums) should be used so that only the cleaning wand, floor tool, and vacuum hose are brought into the patient care area. Central vacuum cleaning systems are most efficiently installed during extensive remodeling or construction of new units.

Cabinet counters, work surfaces, and similar horizontal areas may be subject to heavy contamination during routine use. These areas should be cleaned at least once a day with a disinfectant–detergent and clean cloths; friction cleaning is important to ensure physical removal of dirt and contaminating microorganisms. Surfaces that are contaminated by patient specimens or accidental spills should be carefully cleaned and disinfected; iodophors formulated for environmental cleaning, phenolic compounds, or hypochlorite are useful disinfectants for this type of surface decontamination.

Walls, windows, and storage shelves may be reservoirs of pathogenic microorganisms if grossly soiled or if dust and dirt are allowed to accumulate. These areas—particularly windowsills and other horizontal surfaces—and similar noncritical surfaces should be scrubbed periodically with a disinfectant–detergent solution as part of the general housekeeping program. Aerosols of phenolic or other disinfectants are not reliable for disinfecting hard surfaces; this method is not recommended.

Faucet aerators may be useful to reduce water splashing in sinks, but they are notoriously susceptible to contamination with a variety of water-loving bacteria. Removing aerators periodically for cleaning and disinfection or sterilization should reduce contamination, at least temporarily. Sinks and drain traps are usually heavily contaminated, frequently with the same bacteria that cause infections in patients; epidemiologically, however, these bacterial reservoirs have been implicated only rarely as the source of bacterial infection in neonates. Sinks should be scrubbed clean daily with a disinfectant–detergent; drain traps should not need routine cleaning or disinfection.

Written policies should be established for the removal and disposal of solid wastes. Sturdy plastic liners should be used in trash receptacles; these liners should be sealed before they are removed from the trash receptacles. In patient care areas, trash receptacles should be cleaned and disinfected regularly. Infectious material requires special handling and disposal.

Special housekeeping personnel should be assigned to clean the nursery. If the nursery is small, they may also be assigned to work in the obstetric areas or other clean areas of the hospital (eg, offices, psychiatric services, or elective surgical areas). Housekeeping personnel assigned permanently to the obstetric or nursery areas should wear scrub uniforms, as should other full-time personnel; those not assigned to these areas exclusively should wear clean gowns when entering the areas. Daily cleaning of the nursery should occur when most neonates are not present.

Cleaning and Disinfecting Patient Care Equipment

Incubators, Open Care Units, and Bassinets

After a neonate has been discharged, the care unit used by that neonate should be cleaned and disinfected thoroughly. An iodophor or quaternary ammonium disinfectant–detergent registered by the U.S. Environmental Protection Agency is recommended for this purpose. Manufacturers' directions should be followed carefully. A bassinet or incubator should never be cleaned when occupied. Infants who remain in the nursery for an extended period should be transferred to a cleaned and disinfected unit periodically.

When a care unit is being cleaned and disinfected, all detachable parts should be removed and scrubbed meticulously. If the incubator has a fan, it should be cleaned and disinfected; the manufacturer's instructions should be followed to avoid equipment damage. The air filter need not be discarded each time the incubator is cleaned, but it should be removed and autoclaved weekly or each time the unit is cleaned. Mattresses should be replaced when the surface covering is broken, because such a break precludes effective disinfection or sterilization. Mattresses may be sterilized by heat or gas. Portholes and porthole cuffs and sleeves are easily contaminated, often heavily; cuffs should be replaced on a regular schedule or cleaned and disinfected frequently with freshly prepared mild soap or quaternary ammonium disinfectant–detergent solutions. Incubators not in use should be thoroughly dried by running the incubator hot without water in the reservoir for 24 hours after disinfection.

Evaporative humidifiers in incubators usually do not produce contaminated aerosols, but contaminated water reservoirs may be responsible for direct rather than airborne transmission of infection. Reservoirs should be filled only with sterile water; they should be drained and refilled with sterile water every 24 hours. In many areas of the United States or in hospitals with a central ventilation system, environmental humidity may be sufficiently high to eliminate the need for additional humidification in most cases, and water reservoirs may be left dry. If humidification is necessary, a source of humidity external to the incubator may be preferable to incubator humidifiers, because an external humidifier can be changed daily and the equipment sent for cleaning and sterilization or disinfection.

Tubs

Some labor and delivery units have installed various types of baths for patients in labor. Simple bathtub-like units are probably effectively disinfected by draining, cleaning, and wiping with disinfectant between patients. Units with agitators require cleaning and disinfecting procedures similar to those used for hydrotherapy tanks. It is unlikely that hot-tub units would ever be considered for the use of laboring patients. They are not routinely drained and present great theoretical risks as well as nearly insurmountable obstacles to assuring adequate disinfection.

Nebulizers, Water Traps, and Respiratory Support Equipment

Because nebulizers are easily contaminated, nebulizers and attached tubing should be replaced by clean, sterile equipment (or equipment that has been subjected to high-level disinfection) by established hospital policy. Failure to replace tubing may result in contamination of freshly cleaned equipment. Water traps should also be replaced daily by autoclaved or disinfected equipment. Only sterile water should be used for nebulizers or water traps; residual water should be discarded when these containers are refilled. Water condensed in tubing loops should be removed and discarded and should not be allowed to reflux into the container.

Other Equipment

Cleaning and disinfection or sterilization of equipment should be performed between use on successive patients. Equipment that is used for only one patient should be replaced, cleaned, and disinfected or sterilized according to an established schedule. For many types of equipment, this may be at least once a day. Disposable equipment should be replaced with approximately the same frequency as reusable equipment is recycled. Disposable equipment should never be reused.

Resuscitators, face masks, and other items used in direct contact with neonates should be dismantled, thoroughly cleaned, and sterilized, if possible. Alternately, the equipment may be subjected to high-level disinfection with liquid chemicals or by pasteurization. Equipment such as tubing for respiratory or oxygen therapy should be either sterilized or discarded after use.

Stethoscopes and similar types of diagnostic instruments should be wiped with iodophor or alcohol before use. Tubing, connectors, and jars of suction machines should be replaced daily with cleaned and sterilized equipment.

Procedures should be established to ensure that the neonate warmers used for resuscitation in the delivery areas are cleaned regularly, as well as after each use; they should always be stocked with clean, sterile equipment and supplies, available and ready for use when needed.

Cultures of Environmental Surfaces and Equipment

Routine cultures of equipment after cleaning and disinfection are expensive and time consuming; they should not be a substitute for specific, clearly written, and carefully followed procedures for cleaning and disinfection. Cultures of environmental surfaces and equipment may be useful as part of epidemiologic investigations, however, and an occasional, selective bacteriologic survey of particular patient care areas or equipment may help determine the effectiveness of existing procedures. These studies should be coordinated with the infection control committee and the microbiology laboratory.

Neonatal Linen

Procedures for laundering, making up packs, and delivering linen to the nursery should be established by the medical, nursing, laundry, and administrative staffs of the hospital.

Each delivery of clean linen should contain sufficient linen for at least one 8-hour shift. Linen should be brought to the nursery from the laundry in a closed cabinet that can also serve as the storage unit. If this system is not used, the linen should be stored in specifically designated cabinets in a clean area of the laundry. Traditionally, linen used in the intensive care, intermediate care, continuing care, and admission/observation areas is autoclaved, but the need for this to prevent infections in newborns has not been established by any studies. Autoclaved linen is probably not necessary in normal newborn care areas.

No new garments or linen should be used for neonates without prior laundering. To prevent methemoglobinemia, garments should be marked with nontoxic dyes.

Disposable Diapers

It is acceptable to use disposable diapers rather than cloth diapers in a nursery. No significance of nonsterile diapers in the epidemiology of neonatal disease has been established.

Care of Soiled Linen

An established procedure for the disposal of soiled linen should be strictly followed. Chutes for the transfer of soiled linen from patient care areas to the laundry are not acceptable unless they are under negative air pressure. Soiled linen should be discarded into impervious plastic bags placed in hampers that are easy to clean and disinfect. Soiled diapers should be placed in special diaper receptacles immediately after removal from the neonate; they should never be rinsed in the nursery. All personnel should be aware that handling dirty diapers with bare hands can result in heavy contamination and transient colonization of the hands with microorganisms that cannot be eliminated easily with hand-washing and can be readily transmitted to the next neonate for whom they provide care.

Plastic bags of soiled diapers (reusable or disposable) and other linen should be sealed and removed from the nursery at least every 8 hours. Individuals who collect the bags of soiled diapers or linen need not enter the nursery if all bags are placed outside the nursery. Sealed bags of reusable, soiled nursery linens should be taken to the laundry at least twice each day; sealed bags of disposable diapers should also be taken away at least twice a day.

Laundering

Diapers and soiled linen from the nurseries should not be removed from their sealed bags until they reach the laundry. They should be washed separately from other hospital linen. It is important that nursery linen remain soft. Acidification neutralizes the alkalis used in the washing process and is responsible for the greatest bacterial destruction.

Fatal poisoning has been observed when an antimildew agent that contained a high concentration of the sodium salt of pentachlorophenol was used in the final rinse in a laundry. Similarly, the chemical trichlorocarbanilide should not be used in hospital laundering because it may be harmful.

In order to avoid such potential hazards associated with chemicals or enzymes used in the hospital laundry, the physician in charge should know of all agents in use and should be informed before any changes are made in laundry chemicals or procedures. Currently, there are no legal requirements for testing laundry or cleaning agents for special hazards to neonates. Therefore, caution should be exercised when new laundry or cleaning agents are introduced into the nursery or when procedures are changed.

Resources and Recommended Reading

American Academy of Pediatrics, Committee on Infectious Disease. Report of the committee on infectious disease. 22nd ed. Elk Grove Village, IL: AAP, 1991

American Academy of Pediatrics, Task Force on Pediatric AIDS. Pediatric guidelines for infection control of human immunodeficiency virus (acquired immunodeficiency syndrome virus) in hospitals, medical offices, schools and other settings. Pediatrics 1988;82:801–807

American College of Obstetricians and Gynecologists. Immunization during pregnancy. ACOG Technical Bulletin 160. Washington, DC: ACOG, 1991

Centers for Disease Control. Guidelines for prevention of transmission of human immunodeficiency virus and hepatitis B virus to health-care and public-safety workers. MMWR 1989;38(suppl 6):1–37

Centers for Disease Control. Public Health Service, Department of Health and Human Services. Guidelines for infection control in hospital personnel. Atlanta: HHS publication no. (CDC) 83-8314, 1983

Centers for Disease Control. Public Health Service, Department of Health and Human Services. Guidelines for isolation precautions in hospitals. Atlanta: HHS publication no. (CDC) 83-8314, 1983

Centers for Disease Control. Update: universal precautions for prevention of transmission of human immunodeficiency virus, hepatitis B virus, and other bloodborne pathogens in health-care settings. MMWR 1988;37:377–382, 387–388

Smolen P, Bland R, Heiligenstein E, Lawless MR, Dillard R, Abramson J. Antibody response to oral polio vaccine in premature infants. J Pediatr 1983;103(6):917–919

Vohr BR, Oh W. Age of diphtheria, tetanus and pertussis immunization of special care nursery graduates. Pediatrics 1986;77(4):569–571

CHAPTER 7

MATERNAL AND NEWBORN NUTRITION

Over the past quarter century, an increased awareness of the positive relationship between maternal weight gain during pregnancy and birth weight of the newborn and the recognition of socioeconomic differences in dietary quality and pregnancy performance have heightened concern about the nutritional status of the pregnant woman.

The woman's body mass index should be determined at the initial prenatal visit to allow for preconceptional intervention recommendations if her status is under- or overweight. An individualized goal for weight gain during pregnancy should be set, and any major or potential nutritional risk factors should be identified. The woman should be asked about her food intake, and, if necessary, she may be referred to a registered dietitian or nutritionist for dietary counseling. In addition, educational materials on nutrition that are available from the American College of Obstetricians and Gynecologists, the U.S. Public Health Service, and the March of Dimes may be given to the patient. If economically unable to meet her nutritional needs, the patient should be referred to public agencies or to the Women, Infants, and Children (WIC) program for assistance.

Ideally, each tertiary perinatal care center should have a nutritional counseling program. Dietitians and nutritionists can educate patients at nutritional risk about ways to correct problems that are dangerous to the health of their fetuses and themselves. Specialized programs for a wide range of nutritional disorders should be available to those who need them.

Antepartum Dietary Recommendations

The recommended dietary allowances (RDA) and recommended energy intakes for adolescent and young adult women when nonpregnant, pregnant, and lactating are listed in Table 7-1. These recommendations should be considered a general guide to nutrition in formulating a balanced diet.

Although energy intakes are based on median weights, RDA for nutrients are judged to meet the known needs of practically all healthy

Table 7-1. Recommended Daily Dietary Allowances for Adolescent and Adult Pregnant and Lactating Women

Nutrient (Unit)	Pregnant	Lactating
Energy (kcal)	+300	+500
Protein (g)	60	65
Fat-Soluble Vitamins		
Vitamin A (μg retinol equivalents)	800	1,300
Vitamin D (μg as cholecalciferol)	10	10
Vitamin E (mg α–tocopherol equivalents)	10	12
Vitamin K (μg)	65	65
Water-Soluble Vitamins		
Vitamin C (mg)	70	95
Thiamine (mg)	1.5	1.6
Riboflavin (mg)	1.6	1.8
Niacin (mg niacin equivalent)	17	20
Vitamin B_6 (mg)	2.2	2.1
Folate (μg)	400	280
Vitamin B_{12} (μg)	2.2	2.6
Minerals		
Calcium (mg)	1,200	1,200
Phosphorus (mg)	1,200	1,200
Magnesium (mg)	300	355
Iron (mg)	30	15
Zinc (mg)	15	19
Iodine (μg)	175	200
Selenium (μg)	65	75

Adapted and reprinted with permission from Recommended Dietary Allowances, 10th ed., © 1989 by the National Academy of Sciences. Published by National Academy Press, Washington, DC

persons. Changes in the RDA from those published a decade ago include listing allowances for micronutrients during pregnancy, rather than increments, and separating recommendations for the lactating woman by the length of lactation.

Caloric Intake

It is important to try to balance the benefits of increased fetal growth with the risks of complicated labor and delivery and of postpartum maternal weight retention. The increased demands of pregnancy require on average 300 kcal/d, but the actual caloric intake will vary based on the mother's prepregnancy height and weight (Table 7-2). Weight gain will also vary if the mother is carrying twins. Regardless of maternal weight gain, there is little evidence that caloric intake influences fetal development.

Supplementation

The increased amounts of other vitamins and minerals recommended during pregnancy (see Table 7-1) can usually be obtained through dietary intake, and the routine use of a multivitamin supplement is not necessary. If there are doubts about the adequacy of a patient's diet, however, a vitamin and mineral supplement that provides the RDA can be given safely. It is important to avoid excessive vitamin and mineral intakes (ie, more than twice the RDA) during pregnancy because both fat-soluble and water-soluble vitamins may have toxic effects. For example, less than 8 times the RDA of vitamin A may be associated with fetal toxicity, and large amounts (ie, 10–90 times the RDA) may cause fetal bone deformities. Sufficient amounts of vitamin A are present in the diet, and supplementation is neither required nor recommended. There have been conflicting viewpoints regarding the effectiveness of the preconceptional and early postconceptional use of folic acid in lowering the risk of *occurrence* of neural tube defects. A prospective randomized study of women who have had a previous pregnancy with a neural tube defect indicates that folic acid supplementation reduces the risk of *recurrence* of neural tube defects. The exact dose that has a beneficial effect has yet to be determined.

In its 1990 report, *Nutrition During Pregnancy*, the Institute of Medicine makes the following recommendations regarding supplementation:

Dietary Assessment

Routine assessment of dietary practices is recommended for all pregnant women in the United States to allow evaluation of the need for improved diet or vitamin or mineral supplements.

Table 7-2. Recommended Total Weight Gain Ranges for Pregnant Women, by Prepregnancy Body Mass Index (BMI)* for Singleton Gestation

Weight-for-Height Category	Recommended Total Weight Gain	
	kg	lb
Low (BMI < 19.8)	12.5–18	28–40
Normal (BMI of 19.8 to 26.0)	11.5–16	25–35
High (BMI of 26.0 to 29.0)	7–11.5	15–25
Obese (BMI > 29.0)	7	15

*BMI = [wt/(ht)^2]

Reprinted with permission from Nutrition During Pregnancy, © 1990 by the National Academy of Sciences. Published by National Academy Press, Washington, DC

Iron

For the general population of pregnant women, supplements of 30 mg of ferrous iron are recommended daily during the second and third trimesters. This amount of ferrous iron is provided, for example, by approximately 150 mg of ferrous sulfate, 300 mg of ferrous gluconate, or 100 mg of ferrous fumarate. Administration between meals or at bedtime on an empty stomach will facilitate iron absorption, but taking ascorbic acid with supplements containing ferrous iron does not enhance iron absorption.

Folate

Although routine folate supplementation of pregnant women is of uncertain benefit, a supplement of 300 µg/d may be given when there are doubts about the adequacy of dietary folate. Women who infrequently ingest fruit, juices, whole-grain or fortified cereals, and green vegetables are likely to have low folate intake.

Multivitamin–Mineral Supplements

For pregnant women who do not ordinarily consume an adequate diet and for those in high-risk categories, such as women carrying more than one fetus, heavy cigarette smokers, and alcohol and drug abusers, the Subcommittee [on Dietary Intake and Nutrient Supplements During Pregnancy] recommends a daily multivitamin–mineral preparation containing the following nutrients beginning in the second trimester:

Iron	30 mg	Vitamin B_6	2 mg
Zinc	15 mg	Folate	300 µg
Copper	2 mg	Vitamin C	50 mg
Calcium	250 mg	Vitamin D	5 µg

To promote absorption of these nutrients, the supplement should be taken between meals or at bedtime.

Nutrient Supplementation in Special Circumstances

As mentioned above, supplementation of other nutrients may be desirable for certain pregnant women in the United States. The following are the subcommittee's recommendations for those special circumstances.

Vitamin D: 10 µg (400 IU) daily for complete vegetarians (those who consume no animal products at all) and others with a low intake of vitamin D-fortified milk. Vitamin D status is a special concern for women at northern latitudes in winter and for others with minimal exposure to sunlight and thus reduced synthesis of vitamin D in the skin.

Calcium: 600 mg daily for women under age 25 whose daily dietary calcium is less than 600 mg. To enhance absorption and limit interaction with iron supplements, the calcium supplement should be taken at mealtime. There is no evidence that older pregnant women (ie, those over age 35 years) have a special need for supplemental calcium.

Vitamin B_{12}: 20 µg daily for complete vegetarians.

Zinc and copper: When therapeutic levels of iron (>30 mg/d) are given to treat anemia, supplementation with approximately 15 mg of zinc and 2 mg of copper is recommended because the iron may interfere with the absorption and utilization of those trace elements.

Neonatal Nutrition

Breast milk is the ideal food for neonates, and mothers should be encouraged to breast-feed. In addition to promoting maternal–neonatal interaction, breast-feeding alone can satisfy the infant's nutritional needs for the first 4–6 months of life.

If a mother decides to feed her newborn with formula, the reasons for that decision should be explored in the event that the decision is based on a misconception. Encouragement will sometimes convince a hesitant mother, who may then be able to nurse successfully. If the mother chooses not to breast-feed, however, she should be supported in her decision.

Lactation

At birth, the resistance of the neonatal intestinal tract to bacterial and viral agents is incompletely developed. Colostrum and human milk contain a number of antiinfection factors, including macrophages, secretory immunoglobulin A (IgA), lactoferrin, and lysozyme, that help to protect the infant from infection until the infant's own antiinfective agents are operational. In families with a strong history of allergy, breast-feeding is likely to be especially beneficial, and the ingestion of solid foods should be delayed until the infant is 6 months of age.

Nutritional Requirements

The recommended energy intake is an additional 500 kcal/d. This increment, coupled with fat stored during pregnancy, should provide sufficient energy for adequate milk production. Other allowances are listed in Table 7-1. The precise dietary management of a lactating patient should be determined by her daily milk volume and level of daily activity.

The maternal diet strongly influences the water-soluble vitamin content of the milk. In addition, the maternal intake of large amounts of vitamin D may be reflected in the milk. The mother at nutritional risk should be given a multivitamin supplement, but such a supplement is not needed routinely. Because the iron intake of the mother has little effect on the iron content of the milk, iron should be administered to the mother only if she herself needs it.

Initiation

The successful management of lactation begins during pregnancy. Prenatal care should include discussion of feeding plans and breast care with the patient. The breasts should be examined to determine whether the nipples are inverted or flat; a shield in the patient's brassiere may help to facilitate eversion. The areolar glands provide adequate lubrication during pregnancy and lactation, and the use of special soaps and ointments is not required. During prenatal visits to the pediatrician, the decision to breast-feed should be reinforced and questions answered about the integration of breast-feeding into the total care of the infant in the first months of life.

The mother should be offered the opportunity to nurse her newborn as soon after delivery as possible. She should be allowed to nurse her newborn in any position that she and the baby find comfortable, and she should be guided so that she can help the newborn grasp the breast properly. Enough of the areola (at least ½ inch) should be in the infant's mouth to permit the tongue to stroke the areola over the collecting ductals against the hard palate in the act of sucking. After a brief sucking period of 3–4 minutes, the mother should break the suction by slipping her clean finger into the corner of the infant's mouth. A brief sucking period is then initiated on the second breast. Several opportunities to nurse can be offered during the alert period following birth.

After the mother and newborn have been transferred to the postpartum unit, they should be together as much as possible. When awake, the newborn should be encouraged to feed frequently to stimulate milk production. Usually, it is wise to alternate the side used to initiate the feeding and to equalize the time spent at each breast over the day. By the third day, a feeding may take 10 minutes or more on each side.

Under normal conditions, bottle feedings should not be offered to a breast-fed neonate for the first 2 weeks of life. If the infant's appetite is partially satisfied by water or formula supplements, the infant will take less from the breast, and milk production will be diminished. Water supplements for either the breast-fed or bottle-fed newborn have not been shown to reduce hyperbilirubinemia in the neonatal period.

Monitoring the Breast-Fed Infant

An adequately nourished infant is usually considered to be one who takes at least six feedings per day and sleeps well between feedings. It is also important to be sure that the infant urinates at least six times each day and gains weight over a period of time. The healthy infant may actually feed 12–14 times each day and have a small moist stool with many of the feedings. A physician or nurse should examine the neonate at 10–14 days of age, especially if the mother is a primipara. Failure to regain birth weight by 2 weeks of age in the term infant may indicate a failure to thrive and requires a careful evaluation of the feeding techniques being used and the adequacy of lactation.

Contraindications

Maternal Illnesses. Only after they are receiving adequate therapy and considered to be noninfectious should mothers with active tuberculosis breast-feed their infants. The infant should be examined for infection and provided with appropriate treatment, if necessary.

Cytomegalovirus is excreted in human milk. Mothers with identified primary cytomegalovirus infection should not breast-feed their infants during the acute phase of illness. Mothers who are chronic carriers of hepatitis B virus, as demonstrated by the presence of hepatitis B surface antigen (HBsAg), excrete the virus in their milk and may infect their infant through this route. Prevention of this infection through the administration of hepatitis B immune globulin and vaccine to the newborn (see "Hepatitis B Virus Infection," Chapter 5) will markedly diminish any risk of infection through this route. Mothers who are HBsAg positive should not breast-feed until their infants have received hepatitis B immune globulin and vaccine.

Human immune deficiency virus (HIV) has been found in the milk of a small number of women whose milk was cultured. The relative risk of infection of newborns from this source is unknown (see "Human Immune Deficiency Virus Infection," Chapter 5). In the United States and in other developed countries where formula is safe and readily available, women infected with HIV should be counseled not to breast-feed their infants.

Endometritis or mastitis being treated with antibiotics is not contra-indicated for breast-feeding. Mothers with active herpes simplex virus infections may breast-feed their infants if they have no vesicular lesions in the breast area.

Maternal Medications. Studies of the effects on the infant of most medications taken by a nursing mother have been inadequate. A few drugs are known to be contraindicated in the breast-feeding mother. It is important that the mother discuss the use of medications with her obstetrician and pediatrician if she wishes to continue breast-feeding. In such a case, the infant should be carefully monitored to detect any adverse effect. Oral contraceptives may be used by breast-feeding women once lactation has been established.

Breast Milk Collection and Storage

Many mothers wish to provide their breast milk for their sick or preterm infants, and they should be encouraged to do so. The feeding of maternal breast milk provides the small or ill infant a variety of beneficial hormonal, enzymatic, immunologic, and cellular elements. Although breast-fed preterm infants may gain weight at a slower rate than formula-fed infants, the unique advantages of breast milk balance concerns about the difficulties in achieving intrauterine accretion rates using human milk. There is general agreement that the use of pooled donor breast milk is the least satisfactory regimen for the routine feeding of small or ill infants. Concern about the potential for the transmission of infectious disease has led to the heat treatment of most banked breast milk, reducing its beneficial aspects. In addition, the composition of donor human milk is dependent on the diet, environmental exposure, and life style of the donor, and may present the infant with a risk that is indeterminable.

Mothers with positive results on a test for HIV antibody or HBsAg should not provide milk for their infants because of the risk to other infants. Although mothers who are HBsAg positive may breast-feed their infants after the infants have received hepatitis B immune globulin and vaccine, it is preferable not to use milk potentially contaminated with hepatitis B virus in the nursery.

Women who donate milk for other infants should be interviewed carefully regarding their history of past and current infectious diseases, their use of drugs and medicines, and other factors that may impair the quality or safety of the milk that they provide. Before they are accepted as milk donors, they should be tested for HIV, HBsAg, and tuberculosis. Women whose test results are positive should not be accepted as donors. These tests should be repeated annually for donors who continue to provide milk or who seek reinstatement as a donor. The potential risks should be explained to mothers whose infants are to receive donated milk.

All women who provide milk for infants should be instructed in the proper techniques of milk collection in order to prevent bacterial contamination. Careful hand-washing is critical, and the nipples should be wiped with cotton and plain water before the milk is expressed. The first 5–10 ml of milk contain a large number of bacteria; discarding this portion greatly decreases the contamination of the expressed samples. Although manual expression, when performed correctly, yields relatively clean milk, many women prefer to use a breast pump. All parts of the pump that are in contact with milk should be washed carefully with hot soapy water after each use.

Expressed milk can be refrigerated in sterile glass or plastic containers for 48 hours without an increase in bacterial contamination. If it must be stored for longer periods, it can be frozen in the freezing compartments of refrigerators for 2–3 weeks, or in a deep freeze at 20°C ± 2° for several months.

Frozen milk should be thawed quickly under running water, with precautions taken to avoid contamination from the water, or gradually in the refrigerator at 4°C. It should not be left at room temperatures for long periods, nor should it be subjected to extremely hot water or to microwave ovens. The very high temperatures that may be reached with the latter methods can destroy valuable components of the milk. Once milk has been thawed, it may be refrigerated for up to 24 hours.

There is no consensus on microbiologic quality standards for expressed milk. In general, each milliliter of expressed breast milk contains 10^3–10^4 colony-forming units (CFU) of normal skin bacteria, such as *Staphylococcus epidermidis* and diphtheroids; this milk can be fed to infants with no ill effects. The presence of gram-negative rods in the milk indicates a problem in the collection technique. When there are more than 10^2 CFU of gram-negative bacteria per milliliter, feeding intolerance has been reported, and higher levels have been associated with suspected sepsis. Bacteria levels in the milk can be controlled by heat treatment. Heat treatment, which involves heating the milk to 56°C for 30 minutes to inactivate HIV, leads to a 15% loss of secretory IgA, a 25% loss of lactoferrin and folate, a 75% loss of phosphatase, and total elimination of beneficial cellular elements.

Expressed milk samples are seldom routinely screened for bacterial count. Such screening should be carried out, however, when there are concerns about the expression techniques and when intestinal intolerance of the milk is suspected. When the milk is to be given by continuous infusion at room temperature, thus creating a risk of bacterial proliferation in the container and tubing, the syringe and tubing should be changed every 4 hours.

Institutions storing human milk should refer to the *Guidelines for Establishment and Operation of a Human Milk Bank*, published by the Human Milk Banking Association of North America.

Formula Preparation

Formula selection and control should be physician directed. New formulas should be reviewed by the appropriate hospital committees and the director of the nursery before use. For mothers who intend to nurse their infants, distribution of discharge formula packages should be discouraged. For mothers who intend to feed their infants with formula, the distribution of discharge formula packages should be consistent with the physician's written orders. The physician should write orders for the formula to be used and the amount to be given at each feeding.

Most hospitals now use prepared formula units with separate nipples that are readily attached to the bottles just before use. These units need not be refrigerated; they may be stored in a convenient, clean, cool area. The sterile cap should be kept on the nipple until the neonate is ready to be fed. If there is a special area where nipples are uncapped and placed on the bottle, it should be kept very clean and should be used only for formula preparation. Alternatively, nipples may be uncapped and attached to bottles at the mother's bedside just prior to feeding. The formula and nipple unit should be used as soon as possible, certainly within 4 hours after the bottle is uncapped, and then discarded. If infant formulas are prepared from concentrated liquids or powders, aseptic technique should be used. Aseptic technique involves mixing concentrated liquid or powder with clean water in clean containers using clean utensils. Containers and utensils are considered clean after they have been boiled for 5 minutes and then allowed to cool for 1 hour. Information regarding the risk of using unboiled municipal tap water is not available. Aseptic technique can be most safely carried out in a laminar flow hood, although such a hood is not specifically recommended by formula manufacturers. Aseptic technique is not likely to damage any nutrients in the formulas, whereas heat treatment—especially autoclaving—may caramelize the sugars, reduce the levels of heat-labile vitamins, and decrease the availability of lysine.

For standard formula, including individual variations, there is no need for a formula room. A 24-hour supply of special formula should be prepared in the pharmacy or dietary or formula room if one is available.

Vitamin and Mineral Supplementation

Infants who are breast-fed may show evidence of vitamin D deficiency if their mothers have a low vitamin D intake or little exposure to sunlight, either antepartum or postpartum. If it is suspected that the mother's vitamin D status is not optimal, the infant should receive supplemental vitamin D, 400 IU/d. This is particularly important if the infant is dark skinned or if there is little possibility of significant exposure to sunlight.

Because of the poor passage of fluoride into the milk, infants exclusively breast-fed for more than 6 months should receive supplemental fluoride even in areas with fluoridated water supplies. Formula-fed infants should be given supplemental fluoride if they do not live in an area with a fluoridated water supply. Supplementation should begin shortly after birth.

The iron content of human milk is low, but the bioavailability is high; 50% of the iron is absorbed by infants who are exclusively breast-fed. It is recommended that these infants be given supplemental elemental iron (2–3 mg/kg per day) when they reach 4–6 months of age. Iron-containing formulas containing elemental iron, 12 mg/dl, should be used for all formula-fed infants, and further iron supplementation is not necessary.

Feedings for Low-Birth-Weight Infants

Infants who weigh more than 1,500 g at birth grow adequately if they are fed a regular 67-kcal/dl (20 cal/oz) infant formula designed for full-term infants or their mother's milk, although they retain calcium and phosphorus at rates slower than the fetal accretion rates. Very-low-birth-weight infants are better nourished if they are fed a 67–80-kcal/dl formula especially designed for preterm infants or their own mother's milk fortified by a commercial mixture. Special formulas for small preterm infants contain easily digested and absorbed lipids (15–50% medium-chain triglycerides), additional protein, easily absorbed carbohydrates (glucose polymers and lactose), and enough added calcium and phosphorus to achieve a rate of bone mineralization faster than the rate that can be achieved by means of regular infant formulas or unfortified mother's milk. Sufficient sodium is added to prevent hyponatremia, while additional trace metals and vitamins are included to meet, at least in part, the special needs of the preterm infant.

Human milk has a number of special features that make its use desirable in feeding preterm infants. It contains antiinfection factors, and the triglyceride structure results in excellent fat absorption. The lipase in human milk facilitates fat digestion and supplements the deficient quantity of pancreatic lipase of the preterm infant. The milk does not provide amounts of protein, calcium, and phosphorus adequate to meet the needs of rapidly growing small preterm infants, however. These shortcomings can be corrected by the addition of nutritionally well-balanced and commercially available dry or liquid human milk fortifiers.

Resources and Recommended Reading

Abrams BF, Laros RK. Prepregnancy weight, weight gain, and birth weight. Am J Obstet Gynecol 1986;154:503–509

American Academy of Pediatrics, Committee on Drugs. The transfer of drugs and other chemicals into human breast milk. Pediatrics 1989;84(5):924–936

American Academy of Pediatrics, Committee on Nutrition. Hypoallergenic infant formulas. Pediatrics 1989;83(6):1068–1069

American Academy of Pediatrics, Committee on Nutrition. Iron-fortified infant formulas. 1989;84(6):1114–1115

American Academy of Pediatrics, Committee on Nutrition. Pediatric nutrition handbook. 2nd ed. Elk Grove Village, IL: AAP, 1985

American Academy of Pediatrics, Task Force on Pediatric AIDS. Perinatal human immunodeficiency virus infection. Pediatrics 1988;82(6):941–944

Committee on Nutrition of the Mother and Preschool Child. Nutrition services in perinatal care. Washington, DC: National Academy Press, 1981

Dwyer J. Maternal nutrition in pregnancy with emphasis on adolescence. In: Grand RJ, Sutphen JL, Dietz WH Jr, eds. Pediatric nutrition: theory and practice. Stoneham, MA: Butterworth, 1987:205–220

Gardner SL, O'Donnell JP, Weisman LE. Breastfeeding the sick neonate. In: Merenstein GB, Gardner SL, eds. Handbook of neonatal intensive care. 2nd ed. St. Louis: CV Mosby Co, 1989:238–260

Jacobson HN. Nutrition and pregnancy. In: Walker WA, Watkins JB, eds. Nutrition in pediatrics: basic science and clinical application. Boston: Little, Brown and Co, 1985:373–388

Lawrence RA. Breast-feeding: a guide for the medical profession. St. Louis: CV Mosby Co, 1989

Neville NC, Niefert MR. Lactation, physiology, nutrition and breast-feeding. New York: Plenum Press, 1983:309–311

Sauve R, Buchan K, Clyne A, McIntosh D. Mothers' milk banking: microbiologic aspects. Can J Public Health 1984;75(2):133–136

Subcommittee on Nutritional Status and Weight Gain During Pregnancy, Subcommittee on Dietary Intake and Nutrient Supplements During Pregnancy, Committee on Nutritional Status During Pregnancy and Lactation, Food and Nutrition Board, Institute of Medicine, National Academy of Sciences. Nutrition during pregnancy. Washington, DC: National Academy Press, 1990

Subcommittee on the Tenth Edition of the RDAs, Food and Nutrition Board, Commission on Life Sciences, National Research Council. Recommended dietary allowances. 10th ed. Washington, DC: National Academy Press, 1989

Zlatnik FJ, Burmeister LF. Dietary protein in pregnancy: effect on anthropometric indices of the newborn infant. Am J Obstet Gynecol 1983;146:199–203

CHAPTER 8

EVALUATION OF PERINATAL CARE

Evaluation of perinatal care plays an important role in reducing maternal and infant mortality and morbidity. To accomplish these goals, reviews should be conducted at the institutional, regional, state, and national levels. The process depends on the availability of accurate data and should take the following form:

- Identification of problem areas that require improvement and application of these findings to continuing education of the perinatal care team

- Improvement of local care through a systems approach, with emphasis on the process of risk assessment and management and its effect on the regional delivery of perinatal care

- Provision of standard data for institutional comparisons of outcome and program evaluation, and for studies of comparative epidemiology

- Documentation of the long-term outcome of perinatal care and practices

Evaluation techniques based on data from vital records (eg, matched birth and death certificates) can be informative. However, this technique is inadequate for identifying specific problems at the local level and, therefore, cannot be used to evaluate the quality of care in an institution. Furthermore, it is often difficult for public agencies to provide information on a timely basis. With the advent of automated vital record systems it may be possible to overcome these problems in the future. In addition, a hospital that specializes in the care of a high-risk population may not be directly comparable to a hospital that serves primarily a low-risk one. Williams et al have devised a method to allow each hospital to compare its perinatal mortality statistics with those of other institutions by adjusting for certain risk factors of the population it serves. As mortality rates decline, the evaluation of morbidity becomes increasingly more important. However, as there is no defined end point (as there is in mortality data) the collection and the evaluation of such data are problematic at this time.

Perinatal Data Base

Appendix F, "Standard Terminology for Reporting of Reproductive Health Statistics in the United States," represents the joint efforts of organizations concerned with the statistical uniformity and accuracy of perinatal care data.

In addition to collecting those measures listed in Appendix F, it may be useful in a perinatal care evaluation to collect data on certain characteristics of the mother, the father, the prenatal care provided, the delivery, and the newborn. Following is a partial list of characteristics that may be included in a hospital perinatal data base:

- *Maternal:* Age, gravidity, parity, education, marital status, economic status, race, drug exposure, ingestion of alcohol and smoking, occupational environment, prior pregnancy complications, and the presence of concurrent medical–surgical disease.

- *Paternal:* Age, education, marital status, economic status, race, and the presence of concurrent medical–surgical disease.

- *Prenatal care:* Date and gestational age at the time of the initial visit to the physician, the number and timing of subsequent visits, the type of facility where the visits occurred, the maternal–fetal evaluation methods used, and the medications administered.

- *Delivery:* Nature of initiation of labor, divided into spontaneous and nonspontaneous (induced) groups; the use of monitoring in labor; timing of rupture of membranes; duration of labor; medications administered; and the type of anesthesia administered for delivery. The route of delivery should be designated. Vaginal delivery should be classified as spontaneous or instrumental, and a vaginal birth after a previous cesarean birth should be noted. Abdominal delivery should be further classified as a primary or repeat procedure. The fetal presentation, any obstetric complications, and indication for operative deliveries should also be recorded.

- *Newborn:* Birth weight; gestational age, including method of calculation; sex; Apgar scores; head circumference; length; any anomalies; diagnoses; and autopsy report.

Statistical Evaluation

Uniformity in recording and reporting data is extremely important to intergroup comparisons. Several standard rates and ratios are widely used for evaluation of local and regional perinatal care (see Appendix F). In addition to these, accuracy and completeness of data make it possible to calculate specific perinatal mortality rates for any clinical entity, age, weight, or time period. The denominator must clearly define a population to which the deaths in the numerator belong, and the study period in the numerator and denominator must coincide. Mortality rates of population subsets can thus be determined, as illustrated in the following examples:

Example 1: Clinical entity, maternal diabetes

$$\text{Perinatal Mortality Rate} = \frac{\text{Fetal Deaths } (\geq 500 \text{ g, Diabetic Mothers}) + \text{Neonatal Deaths (Diabetic Mothers)} \times 1{,}000}{\text{Total Live Births (Diabetic Mothers)} + \text{Fetal Deaths } (\geq 500 \text{ g, Diabetic Mothers})}$$

Example 2: Weight-specific neonatal mortality rate

$$\text{Mortality Rate of Neonates } (1{,}000 \text{ to } < 1{,}500 \text{ g}) = \frac{\text{Neonatal Deaths } (1{,}000 \text{ to } < 1{,}500 \text{ g}) \times 1{,}000}{\text{Total Live Births } (1{,}000 \text{ to } < 1{,}500 \text{ g})}$$

Example 3: Age-specific fetal mortality rate

$$\text{Fetal Mortality Rate } (32\text{–}36 \text{ weeks}) = \frac{\text{Fetal Deaths } (32\text{–}36 \text{ weeks}) \times 1{,}000}{\text{Total Live Births } (32\text{–}36 \text{ weeks}) + \text{Fetal Deaths } (\geq 500 \text{ g}, 32\text{–}36 \text{ weeks})}$$

The fetal mortality rate plus the neonatal mortality rate does not equal the perinatal mortality rate, because the denominators are different. The differences, however, are small. These differences may be avoided by expressing each of these with the same denominator (ie, live births).

When there are relatively small numbers in the numerators, the rates or ratios may vary greatly from year to year. It may, therefore, be necessary to perform statistical tests for significance in order to evaluate trends over time.

Hospital Evaluation

The major concern of the practicing physician and the local hospital is to provide the best possible quality care for patients. Regional and national statistics rarely pinpoint local problems; the most meaningful evaluation originates at the local hospital. The process of evaluation at the local level should be simple in design, should involve minimal paper work and maximal visibility, and should provide for input from all members of the health care team. There is no single solution to the problem of local evaluation, but the following suggestions may be helpful.

All clinical information should be recorded on an obstetric and neonatal interim or discharge summary that provides complete information for patient charts, for the obstetrician, for the pediatrician, and for a hospital body charged with concurrent review of care; however, in case of very-low-birth-weight infants the clinical summary may be delayed. In addition, a simple monthly tabulation of delivery and nursery statistics should be available to all staff members of the obstetric and newborn units. Deaths should be recorded on a separate form that shows the date, hospital unit number, name, birth weight, and presumptive cause of death. This allows for regular local peer review.

Periodically the health care team should meet to review summaries and address key questions regarding each death or significant morbidity. This should be done as a standing perinatal morbidity/mortality committee, the membership of which is defined by the hospital's bylaws. However, every effort should be expended to invite those professionals who were involved in the care of the particular patients to be reviewed. Outcome assessment should lead to structure and process evaluation. Ultimately, each event may be classified as potentially preventable or nonpreventable or the care in each situation as appropriate or inappropriate. If the death is classified as potentially preventable in retrospective review, the means of prevention should be identified. If the care is classified as inappropriate, more appropriate care should be defined. The results of such deliberations should be communicated to the chief(s) of service and to those directly involved with the care. Peer review should be viewed as educational rather than as a disciplinary process. Yearly review can provide further critical evaluation as well as be an important learning experience for all members of the health care team. Trends in care can easily be documented by simple tabulation, graphic illustration, and the display of several years of data. Many hospitals are now using computers for the storage, retrieval, and analysis of data.

Quality Assurance

Every hospital should have a quality assessment program to determine whether the provision of care has been effective. Evaluation of patient care should include assessments of the completeness of medical records, the accuracy of diagnoses, the appropriateness of the use of laboratory and other services, and the outcome of care. It should also include the identification of existing or potential problems in the care of patients, the objective assessment of the causes of these problems, and the designation of mechanisms or actions to eliminate them insofar as is possible. The American Hospital Association has issued guidelines to underscore the responsibility for quality assurance, to outline the elements of a program, and to identify ways in which the results should be integrated and utilized to enhance the quality of care.

An evaluation of the use of personnel, finances, equipment, facilities, and length of stay determines the efficiency of the use of medical resources. Each hospital should have a utilization review program to enable proper allocation of its resources without compromising the quality of patient care. There should be a written plan of review, and members of the obstetric patient care team should be involved in the performance of all resource reviews.

Outcome assessment is currently receiving a new emphasis. Clinical indicators are used to direct attention to specific situations in which there is a possibility of unsatisfactory outcome or deficient quality. Structure (eg, equipment availability and physician credentialing) and process criteria (eg, appropriate performance of examinations and tests and accurate recording of results) are then applied to those situations for further evaluation. With this approach, both clinical performance and capability are assured. *Quality Assurance in Obstetrics and Gynecology* is a helpful resource for outcome assessment.

The additional emphasis on outcome assessment in quality assurance and accreditation processes is compatible with traditional individual care of perinatal patients and regional programs. Concepts such as risk assessment and tools such as regional data systems are integral parts of perinatal care and newer directions in quality assurance. The quality assurance process is very dependent on the cases brought before the committee of clinicians for review. A sophisticated departmental or institutional computer system can automate this process once a set of clinical criteria is established to indicate that a case needs to be reviewed. Outcome criteria may include selected maternal, fetal, and neonatal morbidity and mortality indicators. Relatively few indicators may be sufficient to detect problems that may adversely affect the quality of care.

Resources and Recommended Reading

American College of Obstetricians and Gynecologists. Quality assurance in obstetrics and gynecology. Washington, DC: ACOG, 1989

American Hospital Association. Quality assurance in health care institutions. AHA Policy and Statement. Chicago: American Hospital Association, 1981

Schroeder SA. Outcome assessment 70 years later: are we ready? N Engl J Med 1987;316(3):160–162

Williams RL, Cunningham GC, Norris FD, Tashiro M. Monitoring perinatal mortality rates: California, 1970 to 1976. Am J Obstet Gynecol 1980;136(5):559–568

CHAPTER 9

SPECIAL CONSIDERATIONS

Clinical Considerations in the Use of Oxygen

The hazards associated with the administration of oxygen to the premature neonate have been recognized for many years. The prolonged use of supplemental oxygen in neonates of low birth weight, especially those weighing less than 1,500 g, has been associated with an increased incidence of retinopathy of prematurity (ROP, also called retrolental fibroplasia). Short-term hyperoxia has not been shown to increase the incidence of ROP, however. Therefore, when the association between oxygen and ROP was first suspected, many clinicians tried to restrict oxygen use. Although the incidence of ROP decreased with restricted oxygen use, the mortality rate of neonates with hyaline membrane disease increased, as did the incidence of spastic diplegia and other neurologic disorders among premature neonates who survived. Thus oxygen was seen as an effective treatment with potential risks.

Although it appears that vasospasm and ischemia of the retina, particularly of the immature retina, may initiate the vasoproliferative process that leads to ROP, many factors other than simple hyperoxia may play an important role in the pathogenesis of ROP. Apnea, sepsis, nutritional deficiencies, and blood transfusions, as well as prolonged oxygen therapy and ventilatory support (especially when accompanied by episodes of hypercapnia and hypoxia) have each been associated with ROP.

Thus far, it has been difficult to see a clear relationship between the partial pressure of oxygen (Pao_2) in the premature neonate's blood and the incidence of ROP. Retinopathy of prematurity has occurred in neonates who have never received supplemental oxygen, in neonates with cyanotic congenital heart disease whose Pao_2 could never have been greater than 50 mm Hg, and in full-term neonates. Conversely, many small premature neonates have undergone sustained periods of hyperoxia without developing ROP. Some neonates have developed severe changes in one eye with little or no disease in the other. Neonates who have been monitored continuously with skin surface electrodes have developed ROP, even when extraordinary attempts have been made to maintain the Pao_2 levels within a recommended range.

Methods of Oxygen Administration and Monitoring

In an emergency, oxygen in high concentration may be administered by face mask or endotracheal tube to a pale or cyanotic neonate. If the neonate requires supplemental oxygen beyond the emergency period, the oxygen should be warmed, humidified, and delivered via a system capable of regulating the concentration (usually by mixing 100% oxygen with variable proportions of compressed air). These principles apply whether the oxygen is delivered by means of a head hood with continuous positive pressure or by means of a ventilator. A calibrated oxygen analyzer should be used frequently, if not continuously, to monitor the concentration of oxygen delivered.

It is necessary to determine the arterial oxygen tension (Pao_2) in order to monitor oxygen therapy. The neonate's color changes from cyanotic to pink as the Pao_2 increases from 20 mm Hg to 35–40 mm Hg, but it is not possible to distinguish between a Pao_2 of 40 mm Hg and a Pao_2 of 140 mm Hg on the basis of color alone. Intermittent arterial blood gas determinations are simple when the neonate has an indwelling arterial catheter, but they become more difficult when no arterial catheter is in place. Intermittent arterial punctures may be used; however, this technique is not always possible in very small neonates. Arterialized capillary measurements have been used in such cases. These measurements produce fairly reliable estimates of the arterial pH and carbon dioxide pressure ($Paco_2$), but the Po_2 measurements obtained with this approach tend to produce an underestimation of the Pao_2, especially when the values exceed 50–60 mm Hg or when perfusion is compromised.

With the development of transcutaneous techniques of estimating arterial oxygen tension or hemoglobin saturation, continuous monitoring for relatively long periods can be accomplished. The transcutaneous oxygen analyzer allows for continuous arterial oxygen tension analysis, while the pulse oximeter measures oxygen saturation continuously. Neither instrument will determine the actual delivery of oxygen to the tissue, since this is influenced by the hemoglobin concentration and cardiac output.

Transcutaneous oxygen analysis offers a noninvasive method for the measurement of arterial oxygen tension. Creation of a constant vasodilatation by heating the skin causes maximal blood flow with few if any differences between the Pao_2 at the arterial and venous ends of the capillary. The skin oxygen tension then reflects the changes in arterial oxygen tension. Oximetry is the measurement of hemoglobin oxygen saturation in either blood or tissue, depending on the color of the hemoglobin, which changes with the degree of oxygen saturation. To differentiate the light transmitted by oxyhemoglobin in blood from that tissue, the pulse oximeter displays only changes in light transmission due exclusively to pulsatile alterations of the intervening blood volume. It is important to note that the transcutaneous oxygen analyzer measures oxygen tension and the pulse oximeter measures oxyhemoglobin saturation, but neither measures Pao_2 or pH. The accuracy of either type of analyzer must compare favorably with the measured transcutaneous O_2 tension or saturation in an arterial blood gas sample.

In order to make a valid interpretation of results from either instrument, one must be familiar with the oxygen–hemoglobin dissociation curve, which describes the oxygen saturation of hemoglobin at any given Pao_2. It is not a linear relationship. At birth, an increase in Pao_2 above 50 mm Hg will cause a small increase in oxygen saturation, whereas a decrease in Pao_2 below 50 mm Hg will cause a significant decrease in oxygen saturation. Conversely, a small increase in saturation above 90% will be associated with a large change in Pao_2, whereas a similar decrease in saturation below 90% will be associated with a relatively small change in Pao_2. In the normal newborn, as the hemoglobin F content decreases with age, there is a gradual shift in the position of the oxygen hemoglobin dissociation curve to the right. In the sick newborn, who may receive frequent red blood cell transfusions, there will be an accelerated disappearance of hemoglobin F with replacement with hemoglobin A, resulting in a shift of the curve to the right at an earlier postnatal age.

The transcutaneous oxygen analyzer and pulse oximeter have been found to be useful in patients whose clinical condition is unstable and who require frequent changes in the amount of administered oxygen. After 30 days of age, primarily in infants with bronchopulmonary dysplasia, the pulse oximeter appears to be more accurate than the transcutaneous oxygen analyzer. Both instruments require that the patient be adequately perfused and normotensive in order to yield accurate readings. If the infant is having right-to-left shunting across the ductus arteriosus, it is important to know whether the electrode or sensor is located preductally or postductally. The transcutaneous oxygen analyzer electrode should be heated to 42–44°C in order to produce adequate blood flow to the skin. The correlation between arterial blood gases and the transcutaneous oxygen analyzer improves with the higher temperature settings. The accuracy of the transcutaneous oxygen analyzer is best when the arterial blood Pao_2 is 100 mm Hg or less. The analyzer should be calibrated every 8 hours and the electrode moved to another site at least every 4 hours. Electrode placement should avoid bony prominences if possible. Complications associated with use of a transcutaneous oxygen analyzer include blanchable and nonblanchable erythema and skin burns. The response time for a transcutaneous oxygen analyzer is approximately 18 seconds.

The pulse oximeter does not require calibration, since all human blood has essentially identical optical characteristics in the measured red and infrared bands and the electronics of the instrument remains relatively stable. The response time is approximately 6 seconds. Pulse oximetry estimations of oxygen saturation are within ± 5% at higher saturations, but some are less accurate at lower saturations (especially below 85%). The two most common causes of artifacts or abnormal values are movement of the extremity on which the sensor is located and exposure of the sensor to direct, high-intensity light. Other causes include methemoglobinemia; use of different sensors or machines, or both; and placement of the sensor on the same limb as the blood pressure cuff. It is important to remember that hyperoxemia is as important an etiology of long-term sequelae as is

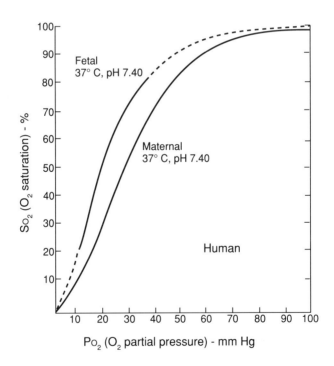

Fig. 9-1. Relationship between O_2 saturation and Po_2 for maternal and fetal blood. (Metcalfe J, Bartels H, Moll W. Gas exchange in the pregnant uterus. Physiol Rev 47:782–838, 1967)

hypoxemia. Because of the shape of the oxygen–hemoglobin dissociation curve (Fig. 9-1), in an infant with a saturation greater than 92%, the pulse oximeter will be less sensitive in identifying an unacceptably high Pao_2. For most neonates, assuming that the hemoglobin content is normal and there is no cardiac failure, an acceptable oxygen content can be maintained with a transcutaneous oxygen analyzer value of 50–80 mm Hg or a pulse oximeter reading maintained at 92 ± 3 (standard deviation), although transient fluctuations out of these ranges may be normal. Individual patients may require different ranges, depending on their clinical situation. If either instrument is used in the delivery room it is important to remember that it may take more than 30 minutes for a normal Pao_2 to read greater than 70 mm Hg or for O_2 saturation in a normal newborn to read greater than 90%. The use of neither the transcutaneous oxygen analyzer nor the pulse oximeter obviates the need for intermittent blood gas analysis. Values should be correlated with an arterial blood gas analysis every 8–12 hours in unstable patients. More frequent arterial blood gas analysis may be indicated for assessment of pH and Pao_2. In stable patients, correlation with arterial blood gas samples can be done less frequently. Both the transcutaneous oxygen analyzer and the pulse oximeter can be used successfully in trending patients to determine the optimal oxygen requirement.

The use of the pulse oximeter and the transcutaneous oxygen analyzer allows for continuous monitoring of oxygen therapy in the newborn. The advantages of continuous oxygen monitoring are that it allows for timely assessment of oxygenation, allows for assessment of trends, and may reduce the need for and frequency of arterial blood gas samples. The disadvantages are that continuous oxygen monitoring tends to replace the use of arterial blood gas samples; adjustments in the fraction of inspired oxygen may be made too frequently, based on guidelines not substantiated by studies; and the transcutaneous O_2 saturation value may be confused with the transcutaneous Pao_2 value. Thus far, there is no noninvasive method for determining the Pao_2 that can completely replace intermittent arterial sampling. If used appropriately, transcutaneous oxygen monitoring may improve the care given to the ill neonate and infant. There should be an institutional policy for documentation of oxygen therapy and monitoring. Current knowledge of the hazards and benefits of oxygen therapy is not complete.

Retinopathy of Prematurity and Oxygen Use

- ROP currently is not preventable in some neonates, especially among those of very low birth weight.

- Many factors other than simple hyperoxia can be important in the pathogenesis of ROP in a given neonate.
- Transient elevations of the Pao_2 alone cannot be considered sufficient to cause ROP.
- There are as yet no standards of care for the use of oxygen that can totally prevent its complications or side effects.

Recommendations

With consideration of the current, but incomplete, understanding of the effects of oxygen administration, the following recommendations are offered:

- Supplemental oxygen should not be used without a specific indication, such as cyanosis, respiratory distress, or a low Pao_2.
- The use of supplemental oxygen beyond the emergency period should be monitored by means of regular estimates of the Pao_2. When this is not possible, oxygen should be delivered in concentrations just sufficient to abolish cyanosis. If neonates delivered before 36 weeks of gestation require oxygen therapy, they should be transferred immediately to a facility with the means to monitor the Pao_2. For more mature neonates, it may be reasonable to administer oxygen for a few hours without such monitoring before making a decision on their transfer. Measurements of blood pressure, blood pH, and $Paco_2$ should accompany that for Pao_2 in neonates who require oxygen therapy. In addition, a record should be maintained of blood gas and ambient oxygen concentrations.
- When supplemental oxygen is administered to a premature neonate, attempts should be made to maintain the Pao_2 at 50–80 mm Hg. Oxygen tensions in this range should be adequate for tissue needs, given normal hemoglobin concentrations and blood flow. Even with careful monitoring, however, the Pao_2 may fluctuate outside this range, especially in neonates with cardiopulmonary disease. It is sometimes prudent to maintain the Pao_2 above 100 mm Hg, especially if attempts to decrease the inspired oxygen concentration dramatically reduce the Pao_2 to very low levels. The concomitantly increased risk of ROP may be unavoidable during such periods. The medical record should reflect the physician's observations, concerns, and decisions relating to oxygen administration, as well as the discussion with the parents about these decisions and the associated risks and benefits.

- Hourly measurement and recording of the concentration of oxygen delivered to the neonate is recommended. The oxygen analyzer should be recalibrated every 8 hours with the use of room air and 100% oxygen.

- Except in emergencies, air–oxygen mixtures should be warmed and humidified before they are administered to neonates.

- An individual experienced in neonatal ophthalmology and indirect ophthalmoscopy should examine the retinas of all premature neonates (ie, those who are delivered at less than 35 weeks of gestation or who weigh less than 1,800 g) who require supplemental oxygen. Infants who are less mature at birth (ie, those delivered at less than 30 weeks of gestation or who weigh less than 1,300 g) should be examined regardless of oxygen exposure. The examination is best done prior to discharge, or at 5–7 weeks of age if the infant is still hospitalized, and should be repeated according to the schedule appropriate to the original findings. Follow-up is recommended for those who have had significant active disease.

Resources and Recommended Reading

American Academy of Pediatrics, Committee on Fetus and Newborn. Vitamin E and the prevention of retinopathy of prematurity. Pediatrics 1985;76(2):315–316

Farrell PM, Taussig LM, eds. Bronchopulmonary dysplasia and related chronic respiratory disorders. Report of the 90th Ross conference on pediatric research. Columbus, OH: Ross Laboratories, 1986

Flynn JT. Acute proliferative retrolental fibroplasia: multivariate risk analysis. Trans Am Ophthalmol Soc 1983;81:549–591

Hay WW Jr. Physiology of oxygenation and its relation to pulse oximetry in neonates. J Perinatol 1987;7(4):309–319

Lucey JF, Dangman B. A reexamination of the role of oxygen in retrolental fibroplasia. Pediatrics 1984;73(1):82–96

Martin RJ, Klaus MH, Fanaroff AA. Respiratory problems. In: Klaus MH, Fanaroff AA, eds. Care of the high-risk neonate. 3rd ed. Philadelphia: WB Saunders, 1986:171–201

Martin RJ, Robertson SS, Hopple MM. Relationship between transcutaneous and arterial oxygen tension in sick neonates during mild hyperoxemia. Crit Care Med 1982;10(10):670–672

Walsh MC, Noble LM, Carlo WA, Martin RJ. Relationship of pulse oximetry to arterial oxygen tension in infants. Crit Care Med 1987;15:1102–1105

Yu VY, Hookham DM, Nave JR. Retrolental fibroplasia: controlled study of 4 years' experience in a neonatal intensive care unit. Arch Dis Child 1982;57(4):247–252

Hyperbilirubinemia

The factors that determine the toxicity of bilirubin to the brain cells of neonates are many, complex, and incompletely understood. They include those that inhibit the penetration of bilirubin into the brain, as well as cell resistance to the toxic effects of bilirubin. In addition, the interrelationships among serum bilirubin concentrations, kernicterus (a condition characterized by a yellow discoloration of the brain with specific yellow staining of the nuclear areas), and bilirubin encephalopathy (brain damage due to bilirubin) in full-term and low-birth-weight neonates are not clear. Yellow discoloration of the brain has been equated with bilirubin encephalopathy in the past, but recent experiments have challenged the theory that they are always associated. The two phenomena may be independent of each other. The incidence of mild neurologic impairment due to bilirubin is not known, nor is it known at what bilirubin concentration or under what circumstances the risk of brain damage exceeds the risk of treatment. Therefore, there are no simple solutions in the management of jaundiced neonates.

Bilirubin Toxicity

A direct association among severe, unconjugated hyperbilirubinemia, kernicterus, and bilirubin encephalopathy has been demonstrated in neonates with erythroblastosis fetalis. In the past, survivors often manifested serious sequelae, particularly the athetoid form of cerebral palsy, hearing loss, paralysis of upward gaze, and dental dysplasia. Observations made some 30 years ago suggested that encephalopathy was unlikely to occur in full-term neonates with erythroblastosis fetalis if serum bilirubin concentrations were kept below 20 mg/dl (342 μmol/L). Subsequent experience in the care of such neonates has justified these conclusions. In other studies, a correlation was found between elevated serum concentrations of bilirubin during the neonatal period and developmental disabilities, but the designs of those studies do not exclude several other causes for the developmental problems. In otherwise healthy term infants, hyperbilirubinemia below 25 mg/dl (428 μmol/L) is not associated with either cognitive or hearing impairment.

Studies of low-birth-weight neonates have failed to identify a specific serum bilirubin concentration as a risk factor for kernicterus. In addition, risk factors such as sepsis, hypothermia, asphyxia, acidosis, hypercapnia, hypoxia, hypoglycemia, and hypoalbuminemia, when present, did not significantly increase the risk of kernicterus at a given serum concentration of bilirubin. In neither of these studies could any single factor or combination of factors (including serum bilirubin concentrations) be associated with an increased risk for kernicterus. These studies underscore the extreme complexity of attempting to correlate serum concentrations of bilirubin and subsequent neurologic status. Nevertheless, there is legitimate concern that subtle neurodevelopmental impairment may represent part of a continuum of neurologic damage associated with hyperbilirubinemia.

With the increasing success of neonatal intensive care, much concern has been expressed regarding the risk of kernicterus in sick, low-birth-weight neonates. As a result of reported autopsy findings of yellow-stained cerebral tissues in premature neonates whose bilirubin concentrations never exceeded 10 mg/dl (171 μmol/L), published guidelines for the management of jaundice in such neonates have suggested early phototherapy and exchange transfusion at bilirubin concentrations as low as 10 mg/dl (171 μmol/L). It has been assumed that, if kernicterus can be documented (at autopsy) at very low bilirubin concentrations, bilirubin-related brain damage may be occurring in some surviving neonates whose serum bilirubin concentrations did not exceed 10 mg/dl (171 μmol/L). Several studies of low-birth-weight neonates have failed to confirm a relationship between serum bilirubin concentrations and later neurodevelopmental handicap, however, particularly if serum bilirubin concentrations did not exceed 20 mg/dl (342 μmol/L). The number of patients in these studies may not have been large enough to detect a small effect, if one existed.

Theoretically, bilirubin must be "free" (ie, not bound to albumin) in order to cross the normal blood–brain barrier. An increase in free bilirubin in the presence of normal or low total serum bilirubin concentrations is the explanation most frequently advanced for the lack of correlation between total serum bilirubin concentrations and autopsy evidence of kernicterus in low-birth-weight neonates. Although there is evidence from animal studies to support this theory, it has not been tested critically in neonates. Furthermore, the correlation between measured free bilirubin concentrations and the presence of kernicterus at autopsy is not consistent. (It is questionable whether free bilirubin actually can be measured, as the methodology is fraught with difficulties. A better term for clinical use is "apparently unbound" bilirubin concentration.) Finally, recent animal studies have provided direct proof that, when the blood–brain barrier is disrupted, albumin-bound bilirubin can color brain tissue. Thus, one possible explanation for the lack of correlation between total (or free) bilirubin concentrations and the development of kernicterus is that other factors (eg, hypoxic–ischemic encephalopathy) alter the permeability of the blood–brain barrier to albumin-bound bilirubin. Whether yellow staining through this mechanism contributes to brain injury is not known.

Management of Jaundice

When carefully reviewed, the data from numerous studies of bilirubin toxicity are so complex that it is difficult to derive a single rational approach to jaundiced neonates. One principle is well accepted: if there is any evidence that a neonate's jaundice is not physiologic, the cause should be investigated prior to the initiation of treatment. Although bilirubin binding tests theoretically may make it possible to determine the risk of bilirubin encephalopathy, they have not yet been validated well enough to be recommended for general use.

Numerous guidelines for the management of jaundiced neonates have been published, but their effectiveness has not been validated by properly designed experiments. Over the past two decades, clinical observations (not experiments) in full-term neonates with hemolytic disease of the newborn have confirmed that the occurrence of clinical kernicterus is highly unlikely if serum unconjugated bilirubin concentrations are kept below 20 mg/dl (342 μmol/L). However, there are no properly designed studies or even observational data in low-birth-weight or full-term neonates without hemolytic disease on which to base clinical guidelines for the treatment of neonates with serum bilirubin concentrations below 20 mg/dl (342 μmol/L). A review of available follow-up data for apparently healthy term infants whose serum bilirubin concentrations were as high as 25 mg/dl (428 μmol/L) showed no apparent ill effects from these concentrations.

Some pediatricians use guidelines that recommend aggressive treatment of jaundice in low-birth-weight neonates, initiating phototherapy early and performing exchange transfusions in certain neonates with very low bilirubin concentrations (less than 10 mg/dl). However, this approach will not prevent kernicterus consistently. Some pediatricians prefer to adopt a less aggressive therapeutic stance and allow serum bilirubin concentrations in low-birth-weight neonates to approach 15–20 mg/dl (257–342 μmol/L) before considering exchange transfusions. At present, both of these approaches to treatment should be considered reasonable. In either case, the finding of low bilirubin kernicterus at autopsy in certain low-birth-weight neonates cannot necessarily be interpreted as a therapeutic failure or equivalent to bilirubin encephalopathy. Like ROP, kernicterus is a condition that cannot be prevented in certain neonates, given the current state of knowledge.

Although there is some evidence of an association between hyperbilirubinemia and neurodevelopmental handicaps less severe than those associated with classic bilirubin encephalopathy, a cause-and-effect relationship has not been established. Furthermore, there is no information presently available to suggest that treating mild jaundice will prevent such handicaps.

Hemolytic Disease

In the presence of hemolytic disease, serial determinations of the serum concentration of bilirubin, not the cord blood concentration of hemoglobin or bilirubin, indicate the appropriate time for the first exchange transfusion (unless the neonate is hydropic or has a life-threatening anemia). The physician may elect to perform an exchange transfusion before the serum bilirubin concentration reaches 20 mg/dl (342 μmol/L), if it appears that the concentration is likely to reach that point. Women who are likely to deliver severely affected, hydropic neonates should be managed in perinatal centers capable of the full range of obstetric and neonatal intensive care.

Breast-Feeding and Jaundice

Many pediatricians have had the impression that breast-fed neonates have higher serum bilirubin concentrations during the first week of life than do bottle-fed neonates. This association of jaundice with breast-feeding, which should be distinguished from true breast-milk-associated jaundice, rests on a body of data that is by no means secure. The composite data from several recent studies reveal that breast-fed neonates have a higher incidence of serum bilirubin concentrations greater than 12 mg/dl (205 μmol/L) than do bottle-fed neonates, however, and the decline in bilirubin concentrations is slower.

There is some indication that frequent feeding (more than seven times per day) may reduce the incidence of hyperbilirubinemia, but supplemental feedings of water to breast-fed neonates do not reduce serum bilirubin concentrations. Furthermore, when an elevated indirect serum bilirubin concentration is due to some pathologic cause, there is no reason to discontinue breast-feeding. The finding of an association between breast-feeding and increased serum concentrations of bilirubin does not imply a causal relationship.

Approximately 1–2% of breast-fed neonates develop the syndrome of breast milk jaundice. The serum conjugated bilirubin concentration rises progressively after approximately the fourth day of life and reaches a maximum concentration of 10–30 mg/dl (171–513 μmol/L) by 10–15 days of life. If breast-feeding continues, elevated concentrations may persist for several days, then decline slowly, and reach normal values by 3–12 weeks of age. If breast-feeding is interrupted at any stage, however, the serum bilirubin concentration declines more rapidly (usually within 48 hours). With the resumption of nursing, the bilirubin concentration may rise slightly, but it does not reach the previous level.

Although no cases of overt bilirubin encephalopathy related to breast milk jaundice have been reported, there have been no prospective studies of a possible relationship in either full-term or preterm neonates. Furthermore, there is no reason to believe that significant elevations of serum bilirubin in the breast-fed neonate are less threatening than are similar elevations in the bottle-fed neonate. If the bilirubin concentration in a breast-fed neonate is rising and seems likely to reach 20 mg/dl (342 μmol/L), nursing may be interrupted for 48 hours. This is usually followed by a prompt decline in bilirubin concentration, and nursing may then be resumed.

Mothers who must temporarily cease nursing should be given positive and enthusiastic support, and they should be encouraged to maintain lactation by using a breast pump or manual expression during the period of interrupted nursing. They should also be reassured that the nutritional value of their milk is not compromised.

Phototherapy

Phototherapy is used extensively throughout the world, and it is an effective means of producing a prolonged reduction of serum bilirubin concentrations in neonates with non-hemolytic jaundice. Exchange transfusion, however, remains the only certain way to decrease the serum bilirubin concentration rapidly and is the treatment of choice when the bilirubin concentration appears to pose an imminent threat to the health of the neonate. Phototherapy is less effective in ABO and Rh hemolytic disease; it reduces, but does not eliminate, the overall need for exchange transfusions. Follow-up studies to date have not demonstrated that the use of phototherapy as prophylaxis in the premature infant or as treatment in the term infant improves neurodevelopmental outcome.

Characteristics of Light Source and the Dose–Response Relationship

Various types of fluorescent light, as well as quartz-halide light, have been used for phototherapy. A minimal irradiance of 4 W/cm^2 in the blue spectrum (as measured by a photometer) appears to be necessary for effective phototherapy. The response increases as the dose increases until a saturation point is reached at approximately 10–12 W/cm^2 per nanometer. Because various instruments provide readouts in different units, caution should be exercised in interpreting measurements from photometers. Blue and green lights have been shown to be very effective; unfortunately, these lights make it more difficult to monitor the true color of infants, and blue light may cause discomfort and vertigo in the nursery staff. A combination of four special blue lamps placed in the center of the phototherapy unit with two daylight lamps on either side has been found to provide excellent irradiance without producing significant discomfort to personnel. Another effective source is tungsten–halogen light. Green light has not been used widely.

Indications

A suggested guideline for the use of phototherapy is to decide on the serum bilirubin concentration at which exchange transfusion will be performed and to initiate phototherapy if the concentration increases to a level 5 mg/dl (86 μmol/L) below that point. In the presence of hemolytic disease, however, it may be appropriate to start phototherapy earlier. In many nurseries, phototherapy is used at much lower bilirubin concentrations, particularly in very small neonates. At present there is no evidence to show that this is either helpful or harmful. If the diagnosis is breast milk jaundice, it is more effective to interrupt nursing temporarily than to initiate phototherapy. Infants who appear to be healthy and who do not have hemolytic disease usually do not require exchange transfusion; thus, phototherapy either in the hospital or at home is rarely indicated for these infants.

Toxicity

Phototherapy has been associated with no known lasting toxic effects in the human neonate. Nevertheless, phototherapy has many biologic effects, and long-term follow-up studies of neonates who have undergone phototherapy are still needed. Because animal experiments have produced documentation of retinal damage from phototherapy, it is recommended that the neonate's eyes be covered with opaque patches during phototherapy. These patches can become displaced and obstruct the nares, however, causing apnea. Appropriate supervision is necessary because of this potential hazard.

Lamp Life

The life of a lamp varies widely, depending on the circumstances and the type of lamp. Overheating in the light chamber causes the phosphorus to deteriorate and shortens lamp life. With adequate cooling, lamp life is usually several thousand hours. In order to ensure lamp effectiveness, however, it is useful to measure the energy output with a photometer.

Resources and Recommended Reading

American Academy of Pediatrics, Committee on Fetus and Newborn. Home phototherapy. Pediatrics 1985;76(1):136–137

Kim MH, Yoon JJ, Sher J, Brown AK. Lack of predictive indices in kernicterus: a comparison of clinical and pathological factors in infants with or without kernicterus. Pediatrics 1980;66(6):852–858

Newman TB, Maisels MJ. Does hyperbilirubinemia damage the brain of healthy full-term infants? Clin Perinatal 1990;17:331–358

Poland RL, Ostrea EM, Jr. Neonatal hyperbilirubinemia. In: Klaus MH, Fanaroff AA, eds. Care of the high-risk neonate. 3rd ed. Philadelphia: WB Saunders, 1986:239–261

Scheidt PC, Bryla DA, Nelson KB, Hirtz DG, Hoffman HJ. Phototherapy for neonatal hyperbilirubinemia: six-year follow-up of the National Institute of Child Health and Human Development clinical trial. Pediatrics 1990;85:455–463

Turkel SB, Guttenberg ME, Moynes DR, Hodgman JE. Lack of identifiable risk factors for kernicterus. Pediatrics 1980;66(4):502–506

Radiation

The National Council on Radiation Protection and Measurements recommends maximal permissible limits for occupational and nonoccupational exposure. These limits are not applicable to medical radiation, however, which is expected to yield a net health benefit to the individual. In attempts to compare the risk associated with medical radiation to other risks in life, it has been estimated that a bone marrow dose of 10 mrads in an adult carries a risk of death of 2 in 10 million, the same risk that driving 3.6 miles in a car carries. The maximal average hypothetical decrease in life expectancy in the United States from medical roentgenograms is estimated to be 6 days; from natural background radiation, 8 days; from motor vehicle accidents, 207 days; and from cigarette smoking by men, 2,250 days.

Maternal–Fetal Exposure

There are three potentially adverse consequences of fetal radiation exposure: teratogenesis, mutagenesis, and carcinogenesis. The single most important determinant of the magnitude of these risks is radiation dose. It is generally accepted that exposure to less than 5 rads is incapable of producing any detectable teratogenic effect in humans or animal models. Bona fide radiation-induced congenital malformations in humans have been reported with exposures in excess of 30 rads, but usually they are seen with exposures of more than 100 rads. The best estimate is that acute exposure to at least 140 rads is necessary to induce a measurable increase in the mutation rate. Diagnostic imaging, including radionuclide studies, expose the fetus to very small doses of radiation. For example, fetal exposure from a maternal chest X-ray is approximately 0.008 rad; from an intravenous pyelogram, 0.400 rad; from computed tomography, 0.250 rad per slice; from an upper gastrointestinal series, 0.550 rad; and from a barium enema, 1.0 rad. Data regarding the risk of cancer in offspring following diagnostic irradiation in utero are conflicting. If there is a risk, it is so small that it is difficult to measure. Exposures will vary based on the patient and the equipment used. If there is a serious question, a radiation physicist should be asked to calculate exact doses. It is very unlikely that even multiple diagnostic procedures could sum to a significant exposure.

Radiation therapy utilizes cumulative doses of 1,000 rads and more. This is an exposure of an entirely different order of magnitude. These doses are capable of causing spontaneous abortion, gross congenital malformation (especially of the central nervous system), microcephaly, mental retardation, and intrauterine growth retardation, depending on the exact dose and timing of the exposure.

Most diagnostic radioisotopic studies are not hazardous to the fetus and involve very low levels of exposure. A typical technetium 99m scan results in a fetal dose of 1–3 rads; a thallium 201 scan, a dose of 0.5–1.0 rad. One important exception should be noted. The fetal thyroid gland begins to trap iodine at 12 weeks of gestation and does so with far greater avidity than does the maternal gland. Therapeutic administration of iodine 131 to treat hyperthyroidism can result in fetal thyroid doses of 1,000 rads or more. It is important to avoid this isotope during pregnancy. Many isotopes are excreted in the urine and can accumulate in high concentration in the bladder. Women should therefore be advised to drink plenty of fluids and void frequently following a radionuclide study during pregnancy.

Ultrasound has obviated the necessity for many diagnostic radiographic studies in pregnant patients. To date, no untoward effects of diagnostic ultrasound have been convincingly demonstrated in humans despite substantial efforts to detect any such effects.

Magnetic resonance imaging involves no ionizing radiation and holds great promise for the future evaluation of maternal and fetal abnormalities, but data are still insufficient to establish its safety and efficacy in the fetus.

It is prudent to minimize fetal exposure to ionizing radiation. Diagnostic radiologic procedures should not be performed during pregnancy unless the information to be obtained from them is necessary for the care of the patient and cannot be obtained by other means (especially ultrasound). When a radiologic procedure is clearly indicated, the radiologist should be consulted to minimize the extent of the procedure and the fetal exposure. There is no contraindication to a diagnostic radiologic procedure that will likely be beneficial to the patient. It is important to discuss the plans for the procedure with the patient so that she understands its necessity and to allay any concerns regarding radiation risks to her embryo or fetus.

Neonatal Intensive Care

Sick newborns require many types of imaging techniques for their care. The skin dose from a newborn chest radiograph is approximately 5 mrads; that from a newborn barium enema, 2.3 rads. Skin doses reflect the maximal dose to the body; as radiation is attenuated internally, doses to the bone marrow and specific organs are lower. There are no data indicating that pediatric patients exposed to numerous diagnostic radiologic studies (eg, premature neonates who have many chest and abdominal radiographs or neonates with congenital heart disease who undergo repeated cardiac catheterization) have a higher incidence of leukemia or other malignancy than does the general population. Nevertheless, because there is a theoretical risk of delayed effects and because young children seem more sensitive to late effects, ionizing radiation is best used only when there is no satisfactory alternative.

Most ultrasound applications in the newborn involve real-time pulse-echo scanning and Doppler studies of fluid velocity. Although ultrasound appears to be safe, it seems appropriate to apply the principles outlined by the American Institute of Ultrasound and Medicine, the National Council on Radiation Protection and Measurements, and the Consensus Development Conference on Diagnostic Ultrasound Imaging in Pregnancy: "Until more is known, it is recommended that diagnostic ultrasound utilization be limited to that extent necessary to obtain sufficient clinical information in each patient. At this time, however, the benefits to patients of use of diagnostic ultrasound appear to outweigh whatever risks may be present."

Abdominal ultrasound examinations are used in a variety of clinical settings in the neonatal period. Such an examination is often the only imaging modality required for evaluation of the solid viscera and major blood vessels. Even when further imaging is necessary, ultrasound findings are valuable in selecting subsequent diagnostic studies. Many neonates in the intensive care unit undergo imaging studies of the brain for diagnosis and follow-up of intracranial hemorrhage. Less frequently, infants undergo such studies for the evaluation of congenital anomalies or trauma to the brain. Three imaging modalities, each with different advantages and limitations, may be used in diagnostic studies of the brain: 1) ultrasound, 2) computed tomography, and 3) magnetic resonance imaging. The energy delivered to the body in the form of sound waves (diagnostic ultrasound) or radio frequency waves and electromagnetic waves (magnetic resonance imaging) has not been demonstrated to cause tissue damage in humans or animals at the power levels of intensity used in diagnostic imaging.

Ultrasound has several advantages in imaging studies of the brain. It uses portable equipment, can be performed rapidly, and does not require absolute immobilization of the patient. The examination can be performed while the patient is in the incubator, which avoids excessive handling and cooling of the neonate. Intraventricular/periventricular hemorrhage, ventricular size, and a variety of congenital anomalies are well demonstrated.

Computed tomography is superior to ultrasound in the demonstration of subarachnoid and subdural hemorrhage, both of which are much less common in the premature neonate than is intraventricular/periventricular hemorrhage. Computed tomography and ultrasound are complementary in the evaluation of cerebral ischemia in the full-term infant. In the follow-up of ventricular shunt placement, ultrasound suffices in many cases; in others, computed tomography may provide useful additional information. The well-collimated fourth-generation computed tomography unit gives a skin dose of approximately 1.4 rads in a standard study of the newborn brain.

Magnetic resonance imaging of the brain in adults and older children has been shown to provide anatomic detail superior to that provided by computed tomography. Its present application to the newborn is restricted by technical considerations, however. For example, magnetic resonance imaging takes more time than does computed tomography. Because the subject must be absolutely still for several minutes, most neonates require heavy sedation before they undergo this procedure. Metal objects, such as respirators and cardiorespiratory monitors, cannot be brought near the magnet, which limits its application for critically ill newborns. On the other hand, studies in stable newborns indicate that magnetic resonance imaging demonstrates fine anatomic detail of the brain parenchyma that cannot be achieved with any other technique.

Personnel

At a distance of more than 1 ft lateral to the primary vertical roentgen beam, radiation exposure to personnel is negligible. Because most neonatal radiography is done with vertical beams, it is generally unnecessary for personnel to leave the room during roentgen exposures. Horizontal beam radiography, used for decubitus and cross-table lateral films, may expose other patients and personnel, however. Care should be taken to ensure that only the patient being examined is in the primary beam.

The strong magnetic field in magnetic resonance imaging units may cause cardiac pacemakers to malfunction and various metallic implants to move. Therefore, personnel who have such devices should not accompany patients to magnetic resonance imaging examinations.

Resources and Recommended Reading

American College of Obstetricians and Gynecologists. Guidelines for diagnostic X-ray examination of fertile women. ACOG Statement of Policy. Washington, DC: ACOG, 1977

American Institute of Ultrasound in Medicine, Bioeffects Committee. Safety considerations for diagnostic ultrasound. Bethesda, MD: AIUM, 1984

Brent, RL. The effect of embryonic and fetal exposure to X-ray, microwaves, and ultrasound: counseling the pregnant and nonpregnant patient about these risks. Semin Oncol 1989;16:347–368

Evans JS, Wennberg JE, McNeil BJ. The influence of diagnostic radiography on the incidence of breast cancer and leukemia. N Engl J Med 1986;315(13):810–815

Laptook AR, ed. Magnetic resonance imaging and spectroscopy. Semin Perinatol 1990;14(3):189–271

National Council on Radiation Protection and Measurements. Biological effects and exposure criteria for radiofrequency electromagnetic fields. Report no. 86. Bethesda, MD: National Council on Radiation Protection and Measurements, 1986

National Council on Radiation Protection and Measurements. Biological effects of ultrasound: mechanisms and clinical implications. Report no. 74. Bethesda, MD: National Council on Radiation Protection and Measurements, 1983

National Council on Radiation Protection and Measurements: Protection in nuclear medicine and ultrasound diagnostic procedures in children. Report no. 73. Bethesda, MD: National Council on Radiation Protection and Measurements, 1983

National Council on Radiation Protection and Measurements. Radiation protection in pediatric radiology. Report no. 68. Washington, DC: National Council on Radiation Protection and Measurements, 1981

National Council on Radiation Protection and Measurements. Radiofrequency electromagnetic fields: properties, quantities and units, biophysical interaction, and measurements. Report no. 67. Washington, DC: National Council on Radiation Protection and Measurements, 1981

National Institute of Health, Office for Medical Applications of Research, National Institute of Child Health and Human Development. Diagnostic ultrasound imaging in pregnancy. NIH publication no. 84-667. Bethesda, MD: U.S. Dept of Health and Human Services, NIH, Office for Medical Applications of Research, 1984

Poznanski AK, Kanellitsas C, Roloff DW, Borer RC. Radiation exposure to personnel in a neonatal nursery. Pediatrics 1974;54(2):139–141

Robinson A, Dellagrammaticas HD. Radiation doses to neonates requiring intensive care. Br J Radiol 1983;56(666):397–400

Shimizu Y, Schull WJ, Kato H. Cancer risk among atomic bomb survivors. JAMA 1990;264(5):601–604

Wagner LK, Lester RG, Saldana LR. Exposure of the pregnant patient to diagnostic radiations. Philadelphia: JB Lippincott Co, 1985

Whalen JP, Balter S. Radiation risks in medical imaging. Chicago: Year Book Medical Publishers, 1984

Yamakazi JN, Schull WJ. Perinatal loss and neurological abnormalities among children of the atomic bomb. JAMA 1990;264(5):605–609

Yoshimoto Y. Cancer risk among children of atomic bomb survivors. A review of RERF epidemiologic studies. JAMA 1990;264(5):596–600

Perinatal Loss

Loss of a pregnancy and neonatal death touches many aspects of a family's life. The intense grief that parents feel about a perinatal death can be confusing and overwhelming. Every effort should be made to determine the etiology of the loss and to understand their grief responses. Effective interventions and management by the health care team, during the mother's hospitalization as well as after discharge, have a critical impact on the parents' ability to adjust adequately to their loss. The goals of the health care team should be to help make the death a reality, to acknowledge the parents' grief, to assure that feelings are normal, to ensure that normal grief reactions begin and are carried through, and to meet the specific needs of individual patients.

Because deaths occur at all levels in the perinatal care system, there should be carefully prepared policies and procedures for the management of families who have experienced a perinatal death. The multidisciplinary aspect of these procedures should be stressed, and the responsibilities of physicians, nurses, social workers, and consultants should be clearly delineated to ensure that the family receives the proper care, support, and information. Such a program of support and counseling has two major components: 1) specific, practical management in the period immediately following the fetal or neonatal death and 2) responsibility for ongoing bereavement follow-up.

Specific practical management in the immediate perinatal period should be directed toward two goals: 1) learning as much as possible about the cause of death and implications for future pregnancies, and 2) helping the parents create a memory of the dead fetus or newborn.

Etiologic Evaluation

When a stillbirth or neonatal death occurs, every effort should be made to determine the etiology so that information can be given to the family. Proper management includes documentation of clinical findings, evaluation of the remains, appropriate laboratory studies, and consultation with appropriate ancillary services. Since there is a bias toward genetic causation with perinatal death, it is prudent to establish a relationship with genetic consultants and laboratories. A thorough diagnostic workup is important and justified for the parents' emotional well-being, as well as for their guidance with regard to future pregnancies. Following is a suggested protocol for this process:

- Prenatal history: This comprehensive evaluation should include a pregnancy history as well as family history of birth defects, pregnancy loss, and neonatal deaths.

- Autopsy: All stillbirths and neonatal deaths should be carefully examined by a pediatrician or other professional familiar with birth defects. These findings should be recorded and communicated with the pathologist who will examine the appropriate tissues. In the case of perinatal death the cord and placenta should be studied. If questions arise because of dysmorphic features, consultation should be considered (if necessary by telephone) with a geneticist or dysmorphologist.

- Photography: Total-body photography is especially important if an on-site consultation concerning dysmorphology is not possible.

- Total-body roentgenograms: It is especially important to obtain X-rays on all cases with limb or other structural abnormalities and whenever disproportion of the fetal/infant body is suspected.

- Cytogenetics: Cytogenetic studies should be undertaken when congenital anomalies or dysmorphic features are present and should be considered on unexplained stillbirths. Chromosomal analysis is also recommended in all cases in which the family history reveals mental retardation, chromosomal abnormalities, unexplained neonatal or perinatal deaths, or multiple spontaneous abortions. Although a sample of heparinized blood can be obtained from the umbilical cord, a peripheral vein, or the heart of fetuses or neonates who have died recently (within 12 hours), the yield of viable white blood cells may be quite small. A more reliable source is a fibroblast cell specimen obtained through sterile procedures up to 48 hours after death and placed in sterile saline, culture medium, or thioglycollate broth. Tissues from macerated stillborns usually will not grow in culture, but tissue from the amnion–placenta may. Care should be taken to avoid contamination from maternal tissue.

- Serology: Serologic tests should be performed for syphilis.

- Frozen liver specimen: Examination of the liver may be helpful when inborn errors of metabolism are suspected.

Autopsy is the only available means of confirming diagnoses and identifying previously unrecognized conditions. It is particularly important in the presence of congenital malformations that may not have been recognized before death but that may recur in subsequent pregnancies. In addition, the autopsy provides an important focus and starting point for follow-up meetings with parents several weeks after a perinatal death. Families who refuse permission for autopsy or who are not approached with this request by their physicians almost always ask questions in follow-up meetings that could have been answered or at least discussed in a more informed manner had an autopsy been performed. The failure to perform an autopsy is frequently due to the physician's benign but mistaken wish to spare the parents further stress or grief or to the parents' misunderstanding of the procedure and its implications. Parents are more likely to consent to an autopsy if approached by the physician who managed the pregnancy or the newborn's care and who understand that by obtaining consent, he or she is taking on the responsibility of seeing that the information obtained is communicated with the family. Parents should have the opportunity to discuss autopsy results face to face. Some preliminary information may be available within several days of the death and should be communicated; however, final results may take several weeks. Parents should be prepared for this delay and told how they will be contacted when final results are available. Copies of the final report should be made available to parents.

Counseling

Bereavement counseling of parents has a very important impact on family members' ability to adjust to their loss and continue with their lives. Each family and each individual react differently to a perinatal death based on their own life experiences (eg, ethnic, cultural, religious background; age; family; and extended family situation) and the circumstances surrounding the death. The health care staff should appreciate these differences. Nevertheless, there are a number of general considerations that hospital procedures can address. One of the most important aspects of care of a mother who has experienced perinatal death is her placement in the hospital during the postpartum stay. The care of these patients is best provided in units where the staff is skilled in postpartum care, has an understanding of the grieving process, and is able to meet the needs of parents experiencing perinatal loss.

In-Hospital Support and Counseling

The time in the hospital after the baby has died is unique in that it is the parents' only opportunity to create a memory of the child. Specific management procedures that assist parents to cope with their grief include:

- Offer the parents an opportunity to see, hold, and spend time with the baby.
- Obtain pictures and remembrances (eg, identification tags, footprints, a lock of hair, birth/death certificates, height and weight records, a receiving blanket of the baby). Even if the parents say initially that they do not want these mementos, they frequently ask for them days, weeks, or months later.
- Encourage the family to name the baby, for it is easier to connect memories to a child if parents can refer to him or her by name.
- Provide information about options for burial, cremation, funerals, or memorial services. Encourage both parents to take an active part in making these arrangements.

- Visit the parents daily while the mother is in the hospital, listen to them sympathetically, and give them information as it becomes available. Physicians should be aware that the staff's potential reactions—guilt, a sense of failure, and uncertainty—may cause them to avoid the parents, thereby impeding discussion of the deceased infant with the family.

- Ensure that the parents have access to support from their families, clergy, and friends. Anticipate with parents difficulties they may have in sharing information about the loss with other children, family, and friends. Provide information and suggestions on how they might handle difficult situations or times.

- Provide reliable preliminary information from the appropriate medical professionals concerning the cause and circumstances of death.

- Explain the grieving process so that the parents understand what the usual reactions are. Parents frequently demonstrate reactions of acute grief, such as somatic disturbances, a preoccupation with the newborn's appearance or probable future appearance, guilt, hostility, and loss of ability to function. Mourning should be allowed and encouraged to proceed.

- Encourage the parents to communicate their thoughts and feelings openly to one another. Help them understand and accept differences in how they grieve.

- Provide written materials for the parents to read in the hospital and after discharge. The period after a fetal or neonatal death always has an element of confusion because of the continuing grief, the tasks of informing relatives and friends, and the need to make final arrangements. Although there can be no substitute for a multidisciplinary group of professionals carefully organized to provide support, written material can provide concrete information about specific procedures, such as autopsy and funeral arrangements, as well as guidance on long-term issues, such as grief, marriage, explanations for young children, and consideration of another pregnancy. These materials can be designed by the individual hospital or obtained through various associations.

- Finally, because families may come from a distance and, thus, may not know their attending physicians well, it is especially important that tertiary care referral centers designate a member of the team who can be an advocate for the family during the hospital stay and following discharge. The designated individual also is responsible for documenting the management and follow-up for each perinatal death. Too often families from afar are lost to follow-up, as physicians, nurses, and families avoid the sadness of bereavement.

Counseling After Discharge

The responsibility for ongoing bereavement counseling depends on the specific circumstances of the death and on the family's relationship to the physician. It is primarily the obstetrician's responsibility in the case of stillbirth and the neonatologist's responsibility in the case of neonatal death to ensure that the family has received counseling.

The ongoing responsibility to the family includes an arrangement for future visits within 4–8 weeks after the death. These visits provide important opportunities for the parents to ask questions and for physicians and nurses to determine whether grieving is appropriate or pathologic. This may be an appropriate time to review the findings of the autopsy and to counsel patients about genetic implications.

Parents should be reassured that loss of appetite, sleep disturbances, loss of interest in sex, spontaneous crying, and frequent thoughts of their dead baby are normal in the grieving process and gradually will become less intense. Referral to bereavement support groups can be very helpful for many families. Pathologic grief is characterized by a more intense and consuming focus on the loss; it may be manifested as an inability to return to work, a loss of interest in self-care and hygiene, severe insomnia, or a desire to stay in bed for most of the day. Individuals who are simultaneously trying to deal with more than one loss or who are in the midst of other family changes may have prolonged or delayed grief. Referral to a psychiatrist, psychologist, or social worker is appropriate for patients experiencing prolonged or pathologic grief. It may be helpful to enlist the aid of the family's pediatrician or school counselor if the other children in the family show signs of difficulty.

To optimize their ability to counsel families that have experienced a perinatal death, hospital departments of obstetrics and gynecology, newborn medicine, nursing, and social services should have an ongoing program of education in the normal grieving process surrounding fetal and neonatal loss. A system of monitoring the effectiveness of this program should also be established.

Resources and Recommended Reading

American College of Obstetricians and Gynecologists. Diagnosis and management of fetal death. ACOG Technical Bulletin 98. Washington, DC: ACOG, 1986

American College of Obstetricians and Gynecologists. Grief related to perinatal death. ACOG Technical Bulletin 86. Washington, DC: ACOG, 1985

Costello A, Gardner SL, Merenstein GB. Perinatal grief and loss. J Perinatol 1988;8(4):361–370

Kochenour NK, ed. Fetal death. Clin Obstet Gynecol 1987;30(2):251–364

Siegel R, Gardner SL, Merenstein GB. Families in crisis: theoretical and practical considerations. In: Merenstein GB, Gardner SL, eds. Handbook of neonatal intensive care. 2nd ed. St. Louis: CV Mosby Co, 1989:565–592

Relationship Between Perinatal Factors and Neurologic Outcome

In the past, the causes of cerebral palsy (CP), mental retardation, and epilepsy were unknown, and they were widely assumed to be due to "brain damage" originating during parturition. This misperception is still held by many physicians, patients, and attorneys. However, it is now known that CP, defined as a chronic motor disability present since early life, is infrequently associated with the events of birth. Mental retardation and epilepsy, in the absence of CP, are not associated with intrapartum events.

Some factors associated with labor and delivery, such as gestational age less than 32 weeks, a sustained fetal heart rate less than 60 beats per minute, breech presentation (not breech delivery), chorioamnionitis, low placental weight, placental complication, and birth weight less than 2,000 g, have a weak statistical link to CP; however, the vast majority of children with these factors do not have later neurologic deficits. Most children with CP have no evidence of perinatal asphyxia.

The term "asphyxia" should be reserved for a clinical context of damaging acidemia, hypoxia, and metabolic acidosis. A neonate who has had hypoxia proximate to delivery severe enough to result in hypoxic encephalopathy will show other evidence of hypoxic damage, including all of the following:

- Profound metabolic or mixed acidemia (pH < 7.00) on an umbilical cord arterial blood sample, if obtained
- Persistence of an Apgar score of 0–3 for longer than 5 minutes

- Neonatal neurologic sequelae, eg, seizures, coma, hypotonia
- Multiorgan system dysfunction, ie, cardiovascular, gastrointestinal, hematologic, pulmonary, or renal system

The term "birth asphyxia" is imprecise and should not be used. (Note: Intrapartum asphyxia implies fetal hypercarbia and hypoxemia, which if prolonged will result in metabolic acidemia. The intrapartum disruption of uterine or fetal blood flow is rarely, if ever, absolute. Terms such as "hypercarbia," "hypoxia," "metabolic," and "respiratory or lactic acidemia" are more precise, both for immediate assessment of the newborn and for retrospective assessment of intrapartum management.)

Only prolonged or severe hypoxia can cause injury to the brain and result in both motor and intellectual dysfunction. Full-term infants with this degree of hypoxia will show signs and symptoms of neurologic dysfunction in the immediate postpartum period. Approximately one third of infants with this degree of asphyxia die. Infants who have been sufficiently hypoxic to cause permanent damage to the brain will show low Apgar scores at 10–15 minutes of age. Evidence of hypoxic cerebral dysfunction will be apparent in these newborns and will include hypotonia, poor feeding, and decreased or absent neurologic reflexes—signs termed hypoxic-ischemic encephalopathy. The severity and duration of these symptoms correlate with outcome. Seizures in the early neonatal period, during the first 36 hours of life, in conjunction with these symptoms are the best predictor of adverse outcome. Apgar scores at 1 minute have no correlation with outcome, and low scores at 5 minutes have little correlation to outcome. Absence of this constellation of findings strongly suggests that substantial hypoxia did not occur during parturition. Their presence does not necessarily indicate that they were due to hypoxia, and other causes should also be considered.

Other markers for alleged birth asphyxia, such as meconium-stained amniotic fluid, abnormal fetal heart rate patterns, low 1-minute Apgar scores, and prolonged labor, in the absence of signs of encephalopathy and seizures have no predictive association with cerebral palsy and occur in a significant percentage of all births.

Although certain nonreassuring fetal heart rate patterns have been associated with low Apgar scores or a low umbilical artery pH, or both, none have been correlated with long-term adverse neurologic outcomes. Therefore, a nonreassuring fetal heart rate pattern alone is not diagnostic of asphyxia sufficient to cause subsequent CP.

Cerebral palsy in low-birth-weight or premature infants is more commonly related to periventricular leukomalacia or periventricular/

intraventricular hemorrhage. The cause-and-effect relationship of these entities to asphyxia is not clear.

Cerebral palsy resulting from severe asphyxia is usually a spastic quadriplegia associated with severe mental retardation. The etiology of the vast majority of other forms of CP is unknown and presumed secondary to cerebral maldevelopment. Preceding neurologic abnormalities may often be the cause of birth asphyxia.

Despite all the technologic changes in obstetrics over the past two or three decades, the incidence of CP remains unchanged in term infants in almost all Western industrialized nations.

Resources and Recommended Reading

American Academy of Pediatrics, Committee on Fetus and Newborn. Use and abuse of the Apgar score. Pediatrics 1986;78:1148–1149

American College of Obstetricians and Gynecologists. Umbilical cord blood acid–base sampling. ACOG Committee Opinion 91. Washington, DC: ACOG, 1991

Blair E, Stanley FJ. Intrapartum asphyxia: a rare cause of cerebral palsy. J Pediatr 1989;112:515–519

Dennis J, Johnson A, Mutch L, Yudkin P, Johnson P. Acid–base studies at birth and neurodevelopment at four and one-half years. Am J Obstet Gynecol 1989;161:213–220

Fee SC, Malee K, Deddish R, Minogue JP, Socol ML. Severe acidosis and subsequent neurologic status. Am J Obstet Gynecol 1990;162:802–806

Freeman JM, ed. Prenatal and perinatal factors associated with brain disorders. National Institute of Child Health and Human Development and National Institute of Neurological and Communicative Disorders and Stroke; NIH publication no. 85-1149. Washington, DC: U.S. Government Printing Office, 1985

Freeman JM, Nelson KB. Intrapartum asphyxia and cerebral palsy. Pediatrics 1988;82:240–249

Gilstrap LC, Leveno KJ, Burris J, Williams ML, Little BB. Diagnosis of birth asphyxia on the basis of fetal pH, Apgar score, and newborn cerebral dysfunction. Am J Obstet Gynecol 1989;161:825–830

Low JA, Muir DW, Pater EA, Karchmar EJ. The association of intrapartum asphyxia in the mature fetus with newborn behavior. Am J Obstet Gynecol 1990;163:1131–1135

Naeye RL, Peters EC, Barthalomew M, Landis JR. Origins of cerebral palsy. Am J Dis Child 1989;143:1154–1159

Nelson KB, Ellenberg JH. Antecedents of cerebral palsy. Multivariant analysis of risk. N Engl J Med 1986;315:81–86

Portman RJ, Carter BS, Gaylord MS, Murphy MG, Thieme RE, Merenstein GB. Predicting neonatal morbidity after perinatal asphyxia: a scoring system. Am J Obstet Gynecol 1990;162(1):174–182

Ruth VJ, Raivio KO. Perinatal brain damage: predictive value of metabolic acidosis and the Apgar score. BMJ 1988;297:24–27

Winkler CL, Hauth JC, Tucker JM, Owen J, Brumfield CG. Neonatal complications at term related to the degree of umbilical artery acidemia. Am J Obstet Gynecol 1991;164:637–641

Substance Abuse

Recent studies have documented that an increasing number of women of childbearing age are abusing licit and illicit substances. Although statistical data are insufficient, there are indications that approximately 1 in 10 infants may be exposed to illicit drugs during pregnancy. The national institute on Drug Abuse 1988 National Household Survey revealed that 8.8% of women of childbearing age admitted to having used an illicit drug in the month before questioning. A recent survey of 36 private and public hospitals showed that approximately 11% of women delivering in these hospitals had used illegal drugs at some time during their pregnancies. A preliminary study in Pinellas County, Florida, demonstrated that cocaine and marijuana use during pregnancy were almost equally distributed across racial and socioeconomic lines.

Drug-Exposed Infants

An increasing number of infants are being admitted to special-care nurseries for complications caused by their intrauterine exposure to alcohol and other drugs. It is important to consider that drug-exposed infants often go unrecognized and are discharged from the newborn nursery to homes where they are at increased risk for a complex of medical and social problems, including abuse and neglect.

The Problem

All illicit drugs reach the fetal circulation by crossing the placenta, and they can cause direct toxic effects on the fetus, as well as fetal and maternal dependency. For example, the opiate-exposed fetus may experience withdrawal in utero when drugs are withdrawn from a dependent mother or, after delivery, when the mother's use no longer directly affects her newborn. Although the incidence of breast-feeding by substance-abusing mothers is generally low, it is important to counsel nursing mothers about the hazards of drug use.

Symptoms of neonatal opiate withdrawal are often present at birth but may not reach a peak until 3–4 days or as late as 10–14 days after birth.

Evidence of withdrawal from narcotics can persist in a subacute form for 4–6 months after birth. Common features of the neonatal abstinence syndrome mimic those of an adult's withdrawal from narcotics. Significant signs and symptoms for the neonate include a high-pitched cry, sweating, tremulousness, excoriation of the extremities, and gastrointestinal disturbances. Although withdrawal from nonnarcotic substances, such as marijuana, does not appear to result in as severe a syndrome of abstinence as withdrawal from narcotics, the newborn may exhibit irritability and restlessness, poor feeding, crying, and impaired neurobehavioral activity also seen in the neonatal narcotics abstinence syndrome. There is a need for increased research to define the degree of permanent residual in these infants.

Environmental factors also place drug-exposed children at high risk for abuse, neglect, and developmental delay. The long-term effects on learning and school performance of children exposed to illicit drugs in utero have not been well documented. Although some research is in press to study this issue, more emphasis is need in this area.

Pediatric Implications

Universal neonatal screening for illicit drugs is not recommended. The long-term consequences, ie, the harms versus the benefits of labeling the infant or the mother (or both), are not known. However, since there are well-documented and potential effects on children exposed to drugs in utero, it is essential that pediatricians recognize drug-exposed infants. Obtaining a thorough maternal history in a nonthreatening, organized manner, from all women, is the key to diagnosis. Screens will surely be negative when drugs were used early in pregnancy and can be negative even when women have taken drugs during the 48 hours before delivery. Because urine toxicology screens may vary among laboratories, pediatricians should be aware that tests for marijuana, its metabolites, and the metabolites of cocaine may not be included unless requested specifically.

Infants and children of substance-abusing parents or guardians are at increased risk for physical, sexual, and emotional abuse. Although all states require physicians to report suspected child abuse or neglect, some states also mandate reporting to child protective services infants with neonatal drug screens positive for illicit drugs. Many of these agencies are overburdened and unprepared to deal appropriately with the potential flood of babies born to substance-abusing mothers. Pediatricians should, therefore, work with their state social service agencies and state legislatures to extend the assistance now available through child protective services. Until that is accomplished, pediatricians should consider recruiting the assistance of the local child protective services agency to provide multidisciplinary treatment and support for the affected mother, child, and family. Local pediatricians should discuss with all professionals and agencies involved how multifaceted problems resulting from drug exposure in utero might best be addressed in their communities. In general, a coordinated multidisciplinary approach in the development of a plan without criminal sanctions has the best chance of helping children and families.

Health Policy

Health policy issues posed by drug-exposed infants can be divided into two components: 1) how to prevent infants from being exposed to potentially harmful drugs before birth and 2) how to address the needs of drug-exposed infants and children.

Prevention of exposure before birth is a vexing problem that has defied solution. At the threshold is a need to explore more effective ways to help people resist the initial and subsequent use of drugs. Until the issue of how to prevent drug exposure appropriately and effectively is resolved, we are left to deal with how to address the needs of drug-exposed infants as children. Although there are some data about the potential for illicit drugs to cause congenital malformations and other health problems in the infant and young child, little is known about subsequent problems confronting drug-exposed infants as they enter their school years and adolescence. Longitudinal studies of these children are crucial.

The following recommendations are offered as a means of dealing with the health policy issues posed by substance abuse:

- Pediatricians can be involved in organizing community-based social service or child protective service systems, designed to provide essential services for drug-abusing women and their children.

- A comprehensive medical and psychosocial history, including specific inquiry regarding maternal drug use, should be a part of every newborn evaluation.

- Newborn urine toxicology should be regarded only as potential adjunct to a thorough maternal drug history. Universal toxicologic screening is not recommended.

- The pediatrician should include maternal drug use in the differential diagnosis of any neonate with suggestive symptomatology.

- The pediatrician should be knowledgeable about state and local child protection reporting requirements.

- In most circumstances, when a drug-exposed infant or drug-abusing mother is identified, the pediatrician should consider recruiting the assistance of local child protective services to provide multi-disciplinary treatment and support for the affected mother, child, and family.

- The pediatrician should evaluate the drug-exposed infant for other medical conditions associated with maternal drug use, including the possibility of concurrent sexually transmitted diseases in the mother and infant.

- Since adverse effects of drug exposure may not be evident at birth, the pediatrician should be alert to potential long-term consequences that may become apparent during ongoing care.

- Models of coordinated multidisciplinary prevention, intervention, and treatment services that improve access to early comprehensive care for all substance-abusing pregnant women and their children should be developed and evaluated. Evaluation of current and new treatment modalities is imperative to determine their effectiveness.

- Funds for research, prevention, and treatment should be made available to address issues of drug-exposed infants.

- The public must be assured of nonpunitive access to comprehensive care that will meet the needs of the substance-abusing pregnant woman and her infant.

- Pediatricians are encouraged to become actively involved in policy issues related to drug-exposed infants and children at the federal, state, and local levels.

Cocaine Abuse in Pregnancy

Cocaine has become a major public health concern as a result of the dramatic increase in its use over the last decade. In the 1970s, cocaine use was primarily limited to the well-to-do because of its expense, with the intranasal route preferred. More recently, there has been a decrease in the street cost and an increasing prevalence of intravenous and smoked routes of administration. This change in the pattern of use has increased the potential for medical complications and for compulsive or addictive use.

Cocaine, with street names of coke, snow, lady, and gold dust, is a local anesthetic derived from the leaves of *Erythroxylon coca*, a tree indigenous to Peru and Bolivia. When administered systemically, cocaine blocks the presynaptic reuptake of sympathomimetic transmitters (norepinephrine and dopamine), allowing for excess transmitter at the postsynaptic receptor sites. The potentiation of norepinephrine results in intense vasocon-striction, an acute rise in arterial pressure, and tachycardia. Both the euphoria and the reinforcing or addictive effects of the drug are thought to be related to the potentiation of dopamine in the central nervous system. Cocaine is commonly used intranasally (snorting), intravenously, orally, and by smoking the free alkaloid form (freebasing). Crack is a highly purified form of the free alkaloid, so named because of the cracking or popping sound made when the crystals are heated in a test tube.

Maternal Implications

The pharmacokinetics of cocaine use during pregnancy has been poorly studied, although cocaine is known to cross the placenta readily. It is thought that urine tests of neonates exposed to transplacental cocaine may be positive for a period of time similar to that for the adult, although benzoylecgonine has been detected in neonatal urine for up to 4 days with an assay sensitive to 10 ng/ml.

Cocaine is degraded by plasma and hepatic cholinesterases to water-soluble metabolites (benzoylecgonine and ecgonine methyl ester). The most commonly used urine test detects benzoylecgonine at a sensitivity of 300 ng/ml. The elimination half-time is approximately 4.5 hours, allow-ing detection in urine for 24–48 hours after varying intravenous doses.

Serious medical complications reported in association with cocaine use include the following:

- Acute myocardial infarction, both with and without underlying coronary artery disease
- Cardiac arrhythmias, including life-threatening ventricular arrhythmias
- Rupture of the ascending aorta
- Cerebrovascular accidents
- Seizures
- Bowel ischemia
- Hyperthermia
- Sudden death

These complications are directly or indirectly attributable to the intense sympathomimetic effects of cocaine.

Research in perinatal cocaine abuse is problematic because of a population of patients who tend to have unplanned pregnancies of uncertain gestational age, to seek prenatal care late, to have suboptimal nutrition, to be heavy cigarette smokers and multiple drug abusers, and to fail to keep appointments. For these reasons, data are often incomplete and control groups are difficult to construct.

As in other substance-abusing populations, cocaine-dependent pregnant women have a high incidence of infectious diseases, especially hepatitis, acquired immune deficiency syndrome, and other sexually transmitted diseases. Other problems during pregnancy are anticipated in a population that underutilizes prenatal care. Even so, cocaine-using women often experience an uncomplicated labor and delivery, although they may be at increased risk of abruptio placentae. The outcomes of pregnancies complicated by cocaine abuse have consistently been shown to be worse than those complicated by abuse of other substances.

Neonatal Implications

Cocaine abuse during pregnancy should be considered a major perinatal risk. Cocaine-exposed infants have an increased incidence of premature birth, impaired fetal growth, and neonatal seizures. Although a specific cocaine withdrawal syndrome in the neonate has not been defined clearly, signs of irritability and tremulousness, lethargy, or an inability to respond appropriately to stimulation may occur. Many, however, seem to have specific clinical manifestations in the early neonatal period.

Perinatal cerebral infarctions have occurred in infants whose mothers have used cocaine during the few days before delivery. These perinatal cerebral infarctions exemplify the severe morbidity that may be associated with intrauterine exposure to cocaine. Issues of increased risk of malformations and abnormalities of respiratory control have been raised but await confirmatory studies. Because most published studies of cocaine's effect on pregnancies and infants have focused on recognized substance-abusing populations, little information is available regarding the effects of low doses of cocaine. In addition, interpretations of clinical studies are complicated by the fact that abuse of multiple drugs often occurs.

A survey of urban hospitals demonstrated positive urine toxicology for cocaine metabolites in 10–25% of pregnancies. The seriousness of perinatal cocaine abuse is underscored by the marked increase in use of the drug by women of childbearing age, by the misconception that cocaine is neither dangerous nor addictive, and by the ability of many cocaine users to hide their habits. Accordingly, the following recommendations are made:

- All pregnant women should be queried regarding past and present drug use at the time of the first prenatal visit.

- A woman acknowledging cocaine use should be carefully counseled regarding the perinatal implications of cocaine use in pregnancy and offered support mechanisms to aid in her abstinence, if appropriate.

- To reinforce and encourage continued abstinence, periodic urine testing for metabolites of cocaine may be desirable in a pregnant woman admitting to cocaine use prior to or during pregnancy. The requirement for consent may vary from state to state.

- Urine testing of the mother or the neonate or both may be useful in some clinical situations, such as in the presence of unexplained intrauterine growth retardation, third-trimester stillbirth, unexpected prematurity, or abruptio placentae in a woman not known to have hypertensive disease, even when cocaine abuse has not been previously suspected.

Resources and Recommended Reading

American Academy of Pediatrics, Committee on Substance Abuse. Drug-exposed infants. Pediatrics 1990;86(4):639–642

American College of Obstetricians and Gynecologists. Cocaine abuse: implications for pregnancy. Committee Opinion 81. Washington, DC: ACOG, 1990

Surfactant Replacement Therapy for Respiratory Distress Syndrome

It is now clearly established that respiratory distress syndrome (RDS) is associated with prematurity-related surfactant deficiency. Since its discovery, there has been a considerable amount of research defining the biochemical composition of surfactant and its relationship to pulmonary function. A considerable amount of research has also been performed on animals to formulate the scientific basis for surfactant replacement therapy in premature infants to prevent or reduce the severity of RDS.

Clinical trials began with the rescue therapy by Fujiwara et al and were followed by several single institution or multicenter trials using bovine, human, or synthetic surfactants. Many of these clinical trials have been published, and others have been submitted for publication. Many of these trials are randomized, and the form of surfactant therapy is either prevention (endotracheal instillation of surfactant at birth) or rescue (treatment after RDS is diagnosed). Based on the published data, it appears that in both prevention and rescue trials, there is early improvement in respiratory status as evidenced by decreased inspired oxygen concentration and mean airway pressure requirements during the first 3 days of life. Some, but not all, published series suggest a reduction in mortality rates and incidence of pulmonary air leaks during the first 28 days of life, but none of the published series appeared to show an improvement in such morbidities as bronchopulmonary dysplasia, necrotizing enterocolitis (NEC), infections, patent ductus arteriosus (PDA), and intraventricular hemorrhage (IVH). In fact, one series showed increased incidence in NEC in the surfactant-treated group, the European trial showed an increased incidence of IVH, and one series showed an increased incidence in PDA in the surfactant-treated group.

In summary, it appears that surfactant replacement therapy reduces the severity of RDS. On the other hand, the evidence that it improves the overall outcome of low-birth-weight infants is still evolving.

The prospect of universal availability of surfactant raises concerns regarding potential misuse of this form of therapy. One such concern is that very-low-birth-weight infants treated by surfactants may stay in nurseries that have inadequate facilities and personnel to care appropriately for infants with multisystem disorders. This is a critical issue since the target population for surfactant therapy is those high-risk, low-birth-weight infants who may have multisystem morbidities that are not beneficially affected by surfactant. Caring for these infants in nurseries that do not have the full ranges of capabilities required may adversely affect the overall outcome.

Following are recommendations for administration of surfactant therapy:

1. The surfactant replacement therapy should be conducted by physicians qualified and trained to do so. Qualifications should include experience in the respiratory management of low-birth-weight infants, including knowledge and experience in mechanical ventilation.

2. Nursing and respiratory therapy personnel experienced in the management of low-birth-weight infants, including mechanical ventilation, should be available on site when surfactant therapy is administered.

3. Equipment necessary for managing and monitoring low-birth-weight infants, including that needed for mechanical ventilation, should be available on site when surfactant therapy is conducted.

4. Radiology and laboratory support to manage a broad range of needs of very-low-birth-weight infants should be available.

5. There should be an institutionally approved surfactant therapy protocol that should be a mandatory component of the quality assurance program.

6. In those institutions in which any of the items in recommendations 2–5 are not present, if an emergency situation arises and if indications are present, the surfactant therapy may be given, but only by a physician who is skilled in endotracheal intubation. Infants should be transferred from such institutions as soon as feasible to a center with appropriate facilities and trained staff to care for multisystem morbidity in low-birth-weight infants.

Resources and Recommended Reading

Avery ME, Mead J. Surface properties in relations to atelectasis and hyaline membrane disease. Am J Dis Child 1959;97:517–523

Enhorning G, Shennan A, Possmayer F, Dunn M, Chen CP, Milligan J. Prevention of neonatal respiratory distress syndrome by tracheal instillation of surfactant: a randomized clinical trial. Pediatrics 1985;76:145–153

Fujiwara T, Maeta H, Chida S, Watabe Y, Morita T, Abe T. Artificial surfactant therapy in hyaline membrane disease. Lancet 1980;1(8159):55–59

Gitlin JD, Soll RF, Parad RB, Horbar JD, Feldman HA, Lucey JF, et al. Randomized controlled trial of exogenous surfactant for the treatment of hyaline membrane disease. Pediatrics 1987;79:31–37

Hallman M, Merritt TA, Jarvenpaa AL, Boynton B, Mannino F, Gluck L, et al. Exogenous human surfactant for treatment of severe respiratory distress syndrome: a randomized prospective clinical trial. J Pediatr 1985;106:963–969

Horbar JD, Soll RF, Schachinger H, Kewitz G, Versmold HT, Lindner W, et al. A European multicenter randomized controlled trial of single dose surfactant therapy for idiopathic respiratory distress syndrome. Eur J Pediatr 1990;149:416–423

Horbar JD, Soll RF, Sutherland JM, Kotagal U, Philip AG, Kessler DL, et al. A multicenter randomized placebo-controlled trial of surfactant therapy for respiratory distress syndrome. N Engl J Med 1989;320:959–965

Kendig JW, Notter RH, Cox C, Aschner JL, Benn S, Bernstein RM, et al. Surfactant replacement therapy at birth: final analysis of a clinical trial and comparisons with similar trials. Pediatrics 1988;82:756–762

Kwong MS, Egan EA, Notter RH, Shapiro DL. Double-blind clinical trial of calf lung surfactant extract for the prevention of hyaline membrane disease in extremely premature infants. Pediatrics 1985;76:585–592

Merritt TA, Hallman M, Bloom BT, Berry C, Benirschke K, Sahn D, et al. Prophylactic treatment of very premature infants with human surfactant. N Engl J Med 1986;315:785–790

Raju TNK, Vidyagascar D, Bhat R, Sobel D, McCulloch KM, Anderson M, et al. Double-blind controlled trial of single-dose treatment with bovine surfactant in severe hyaline membrane disease. Lancet 1987;1(8534):651–656

Soll RF, Hoekstra RE, Fangman JJ, Corbet AJ, Adams JM, James LS, et al. Ross Collaborative Surfactant Prevention Study Group. Multicenter trial of single-dose modified bovine surfactant extract (survanta) for prevention of respiratory distress syndrome. Pediatrics 1990;85:1092–1102

APPENDIX A

Illustrative Categorization of Perinatal Care Personnel and Services

The following matrix is offered as a guide in the functional organization of individual regional programs. The broad goals of a program (ie, reduction of perinatal mortality and morbidity, efficient utilization of resources) should be linked to specific functional services, available education, research, and administrative objectives that are locally determined. Parts of the matrix can be modified according to local needs and resources. The guidelines given here and, in greater detail, in Chapter 1 are probably attainable in most regions.

Table A-1. Perinatal Care Personnel and Services

	Level I	Level II	Level III
		General	
Function	Risk assessment Management of uncomplicated perinatal care Stabilization of unexpected problems Initiation of maternal and neonatal transports Patient and community education Data collection and evaluation	Level I plus: Diagnosis and treatment of selected high-risk pregnancies and neonatal problems Initiation and acceptance of maternal–fetal and neonatal transports Education of allied health personnel Residency education (affiliation)	Levels I and II plus: Diagnosis and treatment of all perinatal problems Acceptance and direction of maternal–fetal and neonatal transports Research and outcome surveillance Graduate and postgraduate education System management
Types of patients	Uncomplicated, emergency, and remedial problems such as lack of progress in labor, immediate resuscitation of depressed neonates, uterine atony, nursery care of large premature neonates (> 2,000 g) without risk factors, physiologic jaundice	Level I plus: Selected problems such as pre-eclampsia, premature labor at 32 weeks and later, mild to moderate respiratory distress syndrome, suspected neonatal sepsis, hypoglycemia, neonates of diabetic mothers, hypoxia/ischemia without life-threatening sequelae	Levels I and II plus: Premature rupture of membranes or preterm labor at 24 to <32 weeks (500–1,500 g), severe maternal medical complications, pregnancy with concurrent cancer, complicated antenatal genetic problems, severe respiratory distress syndrome, sepsis, severe postasphyxia, symptomatic congenital cardiac and other systems disease, neonates with special needs (eg, hyperalimentation), prolonged mechanical ventilation

Personnel

	Level I	Level II	Level III
Chief of service	One physician responsible for perinatal care (or codirectors from obstetrics and pediatrics)	Joint Planning: Ob: Board-certified obstetrician with special competence, special interest, experience, or training in maternal–fetal medicine Peds: Board-certified pediatrician with certification, special interest, experience, or training in neonatology	Codirectors: Ob: Full-time board-certified obstetrician with special competence in maternal–fetal medicine Peds: Full-time board-certified pediatrician with certification in neonatal medicine
Other physicians	Physician (or certified nurse–midwife) at all deliveries Anesthesia services Physician care for neonates	Level I plus: Board-certified director of anesthesia services Medical, surgical, radiology, pathology consultation	Levels I and II plus: Anesthesiologists with special training or experience in perinatal and pediatric anesthesia Obstetric and pediatric, medical and surgical subspecialists
Supervisory nurse	RN in charge of perinatal facilities	Separate head nurses with educational preparation and advanced skills for maternal–fetal neonatal services	Director/supervisor of perinatal services with educational preparation and advanced skills for maternal–fetal and neonatal services
Staff nurse/patient ratio	Normal labor 1:2 Second stage of labor 1:1 Oxytocin induction and augmentation 1:2 Cesarean delivery 1:1 Normal nursery 1:6 Admission nursery 1:4	Level I plus: Complicated labor/delivery 1:1 Intermediate nursery 1:2–3	Levels I and II plus: Intensive neonatal care 1:1–2 Critical care of unstable neonate >1:1

(continued)

Table A-1. Perinatal Care Personnel and Services (continued)

	Level I	Level II	Level III
Other personnel	LPN, assistants under direction of an RN	Level I plus: Social service, Biomedical engineering, Respiratory therapy, Laboratory as needed, Neonatal nurse practitioners	Levels I and II plus: Designated and often full-time social service, Respiratory therapy, Biomedical engineering, Laboratory technician, Ultrasound technician, Neonatal nurse practitioners and clinical specialists, Nurse program and education coordinators
Laboratory (microtechnique for neonates)			
Within 15 min	Hematocrit	Blood gases, blood type, and Rh	Level II
Within 1 h	Glucose, BUN, creatinine, blood gases, routine urinalysis	Level I plus: Electrolytes, coagulation studies, blood available from type and screen program	Levels I and II plus: Special blood and amniotic fluid tests
Within 1–6 h	CBC, platelet appearance on smear, blood chemistries, blood typed and cross-matched, Coombs tests, bacterial smear	Level I plus: Magnesium, urine electrolytes, hepatitis B surface antigen (6–12 h)	Levels I and II

Within 24–48 h	Bacterial cultures and antibiotic sensitivity	Level I plus: Metabolic screening	Levels I and II
Within hospital or facilities available	Viral cultures	Level I	Level I plus: Laboratory facilities available
Radiography and ultrasound	Technicians on call 24 h/day, available in 30 min. Technicians experienced in performing abdominal, pelvic, and OB ultrasound examinations. Professional interpretation available on 24-h basis. Portable X-ray and ultrasound equipment available to labor, delivery, and nursery areas	Experienced radiology technicians immediately available in hospital, ultrasound on call. Professional interpretation readily available. Portable X-ray and ultrasound equipment available to labor, delivery, and nursery areas	Level II plus: Computed tomography. Cardiac catheterization. Sophisticated equipment for emergency GI, GU, or CNS studies available 24 h/day
Blood bank	Technicians on call 24 h/day, available in 30 min, performance of routine blood banking procedures	Experienced technicians immediately available in hospital for blood banking procedures and identification of irregular antibodies. Blood component therapy readily available	Level II plus: Resource center for network. Direct line communications to labor, delivery, and nursery areas

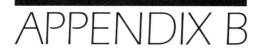

APPENDIX B

Maternal Consultation/Transfer Record

Date of referral call _____ Time _____

Person receiving call _____

Patient's name _____ Telephone _____

Referring physician _____ Telephone _____

Referring hospital _____ Patient Unit _____

Telephone _____ Person calling _____

Reason for admission _____

_____

Maternal History

1. Age _____

2. Gravida _____

3. Para _____

4. Abortion _____

5. Weeks of gestation _____

6. Last menstrual period _____ Estimated date of delivery _____

7. Onset of contractions _____

8. Frequency of contractions _____

9. Cervical dilatation _____

10. Evidence of vaginal bleeding _____

11. Rupture of membranes? Yes _____ No _____ Time _____

12. Fetal heart rate: Infant 1 _____ Infant 2 _____ Other _____

13. a. Temperature _____ b. Blood pressure _____ c. Pulse _____

14. Blood type _____

15. Referral history _____

    Relevant health problems _____

    _____

    Perinatal history _____

    _____

    Reason for transfer _____

    _____

16. Referral plan _____

17. Transported by _____

18. Assessment by _____

    Date _____

APPENDIX C

Newborn Consultation/Transfer Record

Date of referral call _____ Time call received _____

Person receiving call _____

Patient identification

Infant's name _____ Insurance _____

         Last   First

Sex (Circle one)   1. Female   2. Male   3. Other

MD who delivered infant _____ Phone _____
("X" over MD if not appropriate)

Referring MD name _____ Phone _____

Primary MD name _____ Phone _____

Hospital delivered at _____ Address _____

         City   State   Zip

Referring hospital _____ Address _____

         City   State   Zip

Name of person calling _____ Referring hospital phone _____

Birthdate _____   Referring Apgars _____   Maternal history _____

Birthweight (g) _____   1 min. _____   1. Age: _____

EGA _____   5 min. _____   2. Grav: _____

    3. Para: _____

    4. Abo: _____

Other significant information

Referral history (include lab & X-ray results):

Preliminary diagnosis:

Oxygen delivery:	Vent mode	Fluid lines placed? _____				Yes	No
1. Hood/mask	1. Bagging	(Circle all that apply.)			1. Apnea?	___	___
2. Ventilator	2. Respirator		Solution	Rate	2. X-rays taken?	___	___
3. CPAP	4. Other	1. Peripheral			3. Blood cultures?	___	___
4. Other	5. Unknown	2. UAC			4. Antibotics given?	___	___
5. Unknown	0. None	3. UVC			5. OG tube?	___	___
0. None		4. Other (specify)					

House officer assessment
and instructions

Vent Mode/Blood Gas Site					House officer assessment	Yes	No
Time				5. None	1. Temp adequate?	___	___
CPAP					2. Monitoring adequate?	___	___
PIP				Ref temp: _____ °C	3. Blood volume adequate?	___	___
PEEP				Ref dextrostix: _____ mg%	4. Glucose adequate?	___	___
Rate				Ref glucose: _____ mg%	5. Ventilation adequate?	___	___
IiT				Ref HCT: _____ %	6. Sepsis suspected?	___	___
Fio₂				Ref blood pressure ___ / ___	7. Meds appropriate?	___	___
Po₂					8. Other (instructions) _____		
Pco₂				Recommendations:	Type of referral _____		
pH					Date _____		
BE					Assessment by		
Site					(last name only) _____		

Ref temp: _____ °C

Ref dextrostix: _____ mg%

Ref glucose: _____ mg%

Ref HCT: _____ %

Ref blood pressure _____ / _____

Recommendations:

Type of referral _____

Date _____

Assessment by
(last name only) _____

Attending consultant
(last name only) _____

APPENDIX D

Federal Requirements for Patient Transfer

Federal law requires that all hospitals providing Medicare services must follow certain procedures when transferring patients with emergency medical conditions. Failure to follow these procedures can result in a $50,000 civil monetary penalty against both the hospital and the physician. The following procedures must be adhered to.

Determining Whether a Patient Has an Emergency Medical Condition

Any person coming to the hospital emergency room requesting examination or treatment must receive an "appropriate medical screening examination" within the hospital emergency department's capability (including ancillary services routinely available to the emergency department) to determine if the patient has an "emergency medical condition." The statutory definition of "emergency medical condition" is not the same as the medical one. Under the law, it is defined as follows:

> "[A] medical condition manifesting itself by acute symptoms of sufficient severity (including severe pain) such that the absence of immediate medical attention can reasonably be expected to result in placing the health of the individual in serious jeopardy, or serious impairment to bodily functions, or serious dysfunction of any bodily organ or part."

It is important to note that with pregnant women who present themselves to a hospital emergency room, the health of the fetus must also be considered in determining whether an "emergency medical condition" exists.

Special Determination of Emergency Medical Condition for Pregnant Women

The statutory definition also makes specific reference to pregnant women. It provides that an "emergency medical condition" exists if a pregnant woman is "having contractions *and* 1) there is inadequate time to effect a safe transfer to another hospital before delivery; *or* 2) transfer may pose a threat to the health or safety of the woman or the unborn child."

245

An "emergency medical condition" does not exist unless the woman meets one of the two above criteria in addition to "having contractions."

Pregnant Women Meeting the Criteria for an Emergency Medical Condition

If it is determined that a pregnant woman is both "having contractions" and meets either of the two other criteria for an "emergency medical condition" noted above, the physician may *either* provide treatment to stabilize her condition—which means delivering the fetus and placenta—*or* may effect her transfer to another medical facility in accordance with specific procedures as outlined below.

Procedures to Follow for Transferring a Pregnant Woman to Another Medical Facility

The patient may request a transfer, in writing, after being informed of the hospital's obligations under the law and of the risks of a transfer. A patient may also be transferred to another medical facility without having requested a transfer provided that the following conditions are met:

Physician or Other Qualified Medical Person. A physician must certify, in writing, that based upon the information available at the time of the transfer, the medical benefits reasonably expected from the provision of appropriate medical treatment at another medical facility outweigh the increased risks the transfer poses to the individual's medical condition and that of the "unborn child." If a physician is not physically present in the emergency department at the time an individual is transferred, a "qualified medical person" (as yet undefined) may sign the certification described above after consultation with a physician who authorizes the transfer, provided that the physician later countersigns the certification.

Receiving Hospital. The receiving hospital must have space and qualified personnel to treat the patient and must have agreed to accept the transfer. The law provides that specialized facilities, such as neonatal intensive care units, cannot refuse to accept patients if space is available.

Transferring Hospital. The medical records from the transferring hospital must be sent with the patient and the transfer must be made using qualified personnel and transportation equipment. It is important to note that the medical records must include the informed written consent or certification required by the statute (as discussed above) and the name and address of any on-call physician "who has refused or failed to appear within a reasonable time to provide necessary stabilizing treatment."

Enforcement and Penalties

Physicians violating these federal requirements for patient transfer are subject to $50,000 in civil monetary penalties for each violation. Hospitals are prohibited from penalizing physicians who, in complying with this law, refuse to transfer patients.

APPENDIX E

Antepartum Record

DATE _____

NAME _____
     LAST   FIRST   MIDDLE

ID # _____ HOSPITAL OF DELIVERY _____

NEWBORN'S PHYSICIAN _____ REFERRED BY _____   FINAL EDD _____

BIRTH DATE	AGE	RACE	MARITAL STATUS	ADDRESS:
MO. DAY YR			S M W D SEP	

OCCUPATION	EDUCATION	ZIP: PHONE: (H) (O)
☐ HOMEMAKER ☐ OUTSIDE WORK ☐ STUDENT Type of Work	(LAST GRADE COMPLETED)	INSURANCE CARRIER/MEDICAID #

EMERGENCY CONTACT: RELATIONSHIP: PHONE:

TOTAL PREG	FULL TERM	PREMATURE	ABORTIONS INDUCED	ABORTIONS SPONTANEOUS	ECTOPICS	MULTIPLE BIRTHS	LIVING

MENSTRUAL HISTORY

LMP ☐ DEFINITE ☐ APPROXIMATE (MONTH KNOWN)   MENSES MONTHLY ☐ YES ☐ NO   FREQUENCY: Q _____ DAYS   MENARCHE _____ (AGE ONSET)
      ☐ UNKNOWN ☐ NORMAL AMOUNT/DURATION   PRIOR MENSES _____ DATE   ON BCP'S AT CONCEPT. ☐ YES ☐ NO   hCG + ____ / ____ / ____

PAST PREGNANCIES (LAST SIX)

DATE MO / YR	GA WEEKS	LENGTH OF LABOR	BIRTH WEIGHT	TYPE DELIVERY	ANES.	PLACE OF DELIVERY	PERINATAL MORTALITY YES / NO	TREATMENT PRETERM LABOR YES / NO	COMMENTS / COMPLICATIONS

PAST MEDICAL HISTORY

	O Neg + Pos.	DETAIL POSITIVE REMARKS INCLUDE DATE & TREATMENT		O Neg + Pos.	DETAIL POSITIVE REMARKS INCLUDE DATE & TREATMENT
1. DIABETES			16. Rh SENSITIZED		
2. HYPERTENSION			17. TUBERCULOSIS		
3. HEART DISEASE			18. ASTHMA		
4. RHEUMATIC FEVER			19. ALLERGIES (DRUGS)		
5. MITRAL VALVE PROLAPSE			20. GYN SURGERY		
6. KIDNEY DISEASE / UTI					
7. NEUROLOGIC/EPILEPSY			21. OPERATIONS / HOSPITALIZATIONS (YEAR & REASON)		
8. PSYCHIATRIC					
9. HEPATITIS / LIVER DISEASE					
10. VARICOSITIES / PHLEBITIS			22. ANESTHETIC COMPLICATIONS		
11. THYROID DYSFUNCTION			23. HISTORY OF ABNORMAL PAP		
12. MAJOR ACCIDENTS			24. UTERINE ANOMALY		
13. HISTORY OF BLOOD TRANSFUS.			25. INFERTILITY		

	AMT/DAY PREPREG	AMT/DAY PREG	#YRS USE			
				26. IN UTERO DES EXPOSURE		
14. TOBACCO				27. STREET DRUGS		
15. ALCOHOL				28. OTHER		

COMMENTS: _____
_____
_____

GENETICS SCREENING
INCLUDES PATIENT, BABY'S FATHER, OR ANYONE IN EITHER FAMILY WITH:

		YES	NO			YES	NO
1.	PATIENT'S AGE ≥ 35 YEARS			10. HUNTINGTON CHOREA			
2.	THALASSEMIA (ITALIAN, GREEK, MEDITERRANEAN, OR ORIENTAL BACKGROUND): MCV < 80			11. MENTAL RETARDATION			
				IF YES, WAS PERSON TESTED FOR FRAGILE X?			
3.	NEURAL TUBE DEFECT (MENINGOMYELOCELE, OPEN SPINE, OR ANENCEPHALY)			12. OTHER INHERITED GENETIC OR CHROMOSOMAL DISORDER			
4.	DOWN SYNDROME						
5.	TAY-SACHS (EG, JEWISH BACKGROUND)			13. PATIENT OR BABY'S FATHER HAD A CHILD WITH BIRTH DEFECTS NOT LISTED ABOVE			
6.	SICKLE CELL DISEASE OR TRAIT			14. ≥3 FIRST-TRIMESTER SPONTANEOUS ABORTIONS, OR A STILLBIRTH			
7.	HEMOPHILIA			15. MEDICATIONS OR STREET DRUGS SINCE LAST MENSTRUAL PERIOD			
8.	MUSCULAR DYSTROPHY			IF YES, AGENT(S)			
9.	CYSTIC FIBROSIS			16. OTHER SIGNIFICANT FAMILY HISTORY (SEE COMMENTS)			

COMMENTS: _____

_____

_____

INFECTION HISTORY	YES	NO	4. PATIENT OR PARTNER HAVE HISTORY OF GENITAL HERPES		
1. HIGH RISK AIDS			5. RASH OR VIRAL ILLNESS SINCE LAST MENSTRUAL PERIOD		
2. HIGH RISK HEPATITIS B			6. HISTORY OF STD, GC, CHLAMYDIA, HPV, SYPHILIS		
3. LIVE WITH SOMEONE WITH TB OR EXPOSED TO TB			7. OTHER (SEE COMMENTS)		

COMMENTS: _____

_____ INTERVIEWER'S SIGNATURE _____

INITIAL PHYSICAL EXAMINATION

DATE _____ / _____ / _____   PREPREGNANCY WEIGHT _____   HEIGHT _____   BP _____

1. HEENT	☐ NORMAL	☐ ABNORMAL	12. VULVA	☐ NORMAL	☐ CONDYLOMA	☐ LESIONS	
2. FUNDI	☐ NORMAL	☐ ABNORMAL	13. VAGINA	☐ NORMAL	☐ INFLAMMATION	☐ DISCHARGE	
3. TEETH	☐ NORMAL	☐ ABNORMAL	14. CERVIX	☐ NORMAL	☐ INFLAMMATION	☐ LESIONS	
4. THYROID	☐ NORMAL	☐ ABNORMAL	15. UTERUS	☐ NORMAL	☐ ABNORMAL	☐ FIBROIDS	
5. BREASTS	☐ NORMAL	☐ ABNORMAL	16. ADNEXA	☐ NORMAL	☐ MASS		
6. LUNGS	☐ NORMAL	☐ ABNORMAL	17. RECTUM	☐ NORMAL	☐ ABNORMAL		
7. HEART	☐ NORMAL	☐ ABNORMAL	18. DIAGONAL CONJUGATE	☐ REACHED	☐ NO	_____ CM	
8. ABDOMEN	☐ NORMAL	☐ ABNORMAL	19. SPINES	☐ AVERAGE	☐ PROMINENT	☐ BLUNT	
9. EXTREMITIES	☐ NORMAL	☐ ABNORMAL	20. SACRUM	☐ CONCAVE	☐ STRAIGHT	☐ ANTERIOR	
10. SKIN	☐ NORMAL	☐ ABNORMAL	21. ARCH	☐ NORMAL	☐ WIDE	☐ NARROW	
11. LYMPH NODES	☐ NORMAL	☐ ABNORMAL	22. GYNECOID PELVIC TYPE	☐ YES	☐ NO		

COMMENTS (Number and explain abnormals): _____

_____

_____ EXAM BY _____

NAME _____
LAST   FIRST   MIDDLE

DRUG ALLERGY:

ANESTHESIA CONSULT PLANNED   ☐ YES   ☐ NO

PROBLEMS/PLANS	MEDICATION LIST:	Start date	Stop date
1.	1.		
2.	2.		
3.	3.		
4.	4.		

EDD CONFIRMATION

INITIAL EDD:		**18–20-WEEK EDD UPDATE:**	
LMP ____ / ____ / ____ = EDD ____ / ____ / ____		QUICKENING ____ / ____ / ____ + 22 WKS = ____ / ____ / ____	
INITIAL EXAM ____ / ____ / ____ = ____ WKS = EDD ____ / ____ / ____		FUNDAL HT. AT UMBIL. ____ / ____ / ____ + 20 WKS = ____ / ____ / ____	
ULTRASOUND ____ / ____ / ____ = ____ WKS = EDD ____ / ____ / ____		FHT W/FETOSCOPE ____ / ____ / ____ + 20 WKS = ____ / ____ / ____	
INITIAL EDD ____ / ____ / ____ INITIALED BY _____		ULTRASOUND ____ / ____ / ____ = ____ WKS = ____ / ____ / ____	
		FINAL EDD ____ / ____ / ____ INITIALED BY _____	

32–34-WEEK EDD–UTERINE SIZE CONCORDANCE (± 4 OR MORE CM SUGGESTS THE NEED FOR ULTRASOUND EVALUATION)

VISIT DATE (YEAR _____)														
WEEKS GEST. (BEST EST.)														
FUNDAL HEIGHT (CM)														
FHR PRESENT: F=FETOSCOPE D=DOPTONE														
FETAL MOVEMENT: +=PRESENT O=ABSENT														
PREMATURITY: SIGNS/SYMPTOMS:* +=PRESENT O=ABSENT														
CERVIX EXAM (DIL./EFF./STA.)														
BLOOD PRESSURE: — INITIAL														
BLOOD PRESSURE: — REPEAT														
EDEMA +=PRESENT O=ABSENT														
WEIGHT (PREPREG: _____)														
CUMULATIVE WEIGHT GAIN														
URINE (GLUCOSE/ ALBUMIN/KETONES)														
NEXT APPOINTMENT														
PROVIDER (INITIALS)														
TEST REMINDERS	8–18 WEEKS CVS/AMNIO/MSAFP			24–28 WEEKS GLUCOSE SCREEN/Rhig										

COMMENTS: _____
_____
_____
_____

*For example: vaginal bleeding, discharge, cramps, contractions, pelvic pressure.

LABORATORY AND EDUCATION

INITIAL LABS	DATE	RESULT	REVIEWED
BLOOD TYPE	/ /	A B AB O	
Rh TYPE	/ /		
ANTIBODY SCREEN	/ /		
HCT/HGB	/ /	_____ % _____ g/dl	
PAP SMEAR	/ /	NORMAL / ABNORMAL / _____	
RUBELLA	/ /		
VDRL	/ /		
GC	/ /		
URINE CULTURE/SCREEN	/ /		
HBsAg	/ /		

COMMENTS/ADDITIONAL LAB

8–18-WEEK LABS (WHEN INDICATED)	DATE	RESULT
ULTRASOUND	/ /	
MSAFP	/ /	_____MOM
AMNIO/CVS	/ /	
KARYOTYPE	/ /	46, XX OR 46, XY / OTHER_____
ALPHA-FETOPROTEIN	/ /	NORMAL_____ ABNORMAL_____

24–28-WEEK LABS (WHEN INDICATED)	DATE	RESULT
HCT/HGB	/ /	_____ % _____ g/dl
DIABETES SCREEN	/ /	1 HR _____
GTT (IF SCREEN ABNORMAL)	/ /	_____FBS _____1 HR
		_____2 HR _____3 HR
Rh ANTIBODY SCREEN	/ /	
Rhig GIVEN (28 WKS)	/ /	SIGNATURE _____

32–36-WEEK LABS (WHEN INDICATED)	DATE	RESULT
ULTRASOUND	/ /	
VDRL	/ /	
GC	/ /	
HCT/HGB	/ /	_____ % _____ g/dl

OPTIONAL LAB (HIGH-RISK GROUPS)	DATE	RESULT
HIV	/ /	
HGB ELECTROPHORESIS	/ /	AA AS SS AC SC AF ↑A$_2$
CHLAMYDIA	/ /	
OTHER	/ /	

PLANS/EDUCATION (COUNSELED ☐)

☐ ANESTHESIA PLANS _____

☐ TOXOPLASMOSIS PRECAUTIONS (CATS/RAW MEAT) _____

☐ CHILDBIRTH CLASSES _____

☐ PHYSICAL ACTIVITY _____

☐ PREMATURE LABOR SIGNS _____

☐ NUTRITION COUNSELING _____

☐ BREAST OR BOTTLE FEEDING _____

☐ NEWBORN CAR SEAT _____

☐ POSTPARTUM BIRTH CONTROL _____

☐ ENVIRONMENTAL/WORK HAZARDS _____

☐ TUBAL STERILIZATION _____

☐ VBAC COUNSELING _____

☐ CIRCUMCISION _____

☐ TRAVEL _____

REQUESTS _____

_____

_____

TUBAL STERILIZATION   DATE   INITIALS

CONSENT SIGNED   ___/___/___   _____

APPENDIX F

Standard Terminology for Reporting of Reproductive Health Statistics in the United States

The definitions, formulae, and reporting requirements presented here were prepared, reviewed, and approved by representatives of the American Academy of Pediatrics, the American College of Obstetricians and Gynecologists, the American Medical Association, the American Medical Record Association, the Association of Maternal and Child Health Programs, the Association for Vital Records and Health Statistics, the Centers for Disease Control, the National Center for Health Statistics, and the Office of Maternal and Child Health to promote uniform collection procedures and the proper use and interpretation of reproductive health statistics.

We believe that the adoption of these recommended definitions and reporting requirements will provide an improved basis for standardization and uniformity in the design, implementation, and evaluation of intervention strategies. The reduction of maternal and infant mortality and the improvement of the health of our nation's mothers and infants is our ultimate goal. The collection and analysis of reliable statistical data are an essential part of in-depth investigations which incorporate casefinding, individual review and analysis of risk factors. These studies could then yield valuable clinical information for practitioners to aid them in improved case management for high risk patients, resulting in decreased morbidity and mortality.

This standardization represents an attempt to enhance communication between those in the medical community who provide the data, those who are responsible for collecting the data, and those who analyze and interpret the data to plan and evaluate perinatal programs.

Both collection and use of statistics have been hampered by lack of understanding of differences in *definitions, statistical tabulations,* and *reporting requirements* among state, national, and international bodies. Misapplication and misinterpretation of data may lead to erroneous comparisons and conclusions. For example, specific requirements for reporting of fetal deaths have frequently been misinterpreted as implying a weight or gestational age for viability. Distinctions can and should be made among 1) the definition of an event, 2) the reporting requirements for the event, and 3) the statistical tabulation and interpretation of the data. The

253

definition indicates the meaning of a term (for example, live birth, fetal death, or maternal death). A reporting requirement is that part of the defined event for which reporting is mandatory or desired. Statistical tabulations connote the presentation of data for the purpose of analysis and interpretation of existing and future conditions. The data should be collected in a manner that will allow them to be presented in different ways for different users. Adjustments should be made for variations in reporting before comparisons among data are attempted.

If information is collected and presented in a standardized manner, comparisons between the new data and the data obtained by previous reporting requirements can be delineated clearly and can contribute to improved public understanding of reproductive health statistics.

For ease in assimilating this information, it is divided into three sections: definitions, statistical tabulations, and reporting requirements/recommendations. Some of the definitions and recommendations are a departure from those currently or historically accepted; however, these recommendations were agreed upon by the interorganizational group that was brought together to review terminology related to reproductive health issues.

Definitions

Live Birth

The complete expulsion or extraction from the mother of a product of human conception, irrespective of the duration of pregnancy, which, after such expulsion or extraction, breathes or shows any other evidence of life, such as beating of the heart, pulsation of the umbilical cord, or definite movement of voluntary muscles whether or not the umbilical cord has been cut or the placenta is attached. Heartbeats are to be distinguished from transient cardiac contractions; respirations are to be distinguished from fleeting respiratory efforts or gasps.

Birth Weight

The weight of a neonate determined immediately after delivery or as soon thereafter as feasible. It should be expressed to the nearest gram.

Gestational Age

The number of completed weeks that have elapsed between the first day of the last normal menstrual period (not the presumed time of conception) and the date of delivery, irrespective of whether the gestation results in a live birth or a fetal death.

Neonate

Low Birth Weight. Any neonate, regardless of gestational age, whose weight at birth is less than 2,500 g.

Preterm.* Any neonate whose birth occurs through the end of the last day of the 37th week (259th day), following onset of the last menstrual period.

Term. * Any neonate whose birth occurs from the beginning of the first day (260th day) of the 38th week, through the end of the last day of the 42nd week (294th day), following the onset of the last menstrual period (Fig. A-1).

Postterm. Any neonate whose birth occurs from the beginning of the first day (295th day) of the 43rd week following onset of the last menstrual period.

Fetal Death

Death prior to the complete expulsion or extraction from the mother of a product of human conception, fetus and placenta, irrespective of the duration of pregnancy; the death is indicated by the fact that, after such expulsion or extraction, the fetus does not breathe or show any other evidence of life, such as beating of the heart, pulsation of the umbilical cord, or definite movement of voluntary muscles. Heartbeats are to be distinguished from transient cardiac contractions; respirations are to be distinguished from fleeting respiratory efforts or gasps. This definition excludes induced terminations of pregnancy.

Neonatal Death

Death of a liveborn neonate before the neonate becomes 28 days old (up to and including 27 days, 23 hours, 59 minutes from the moment of birth).

---

*These definitions are for statistical purposes and not intended to affect clinical management. Appropriate assessment of fetal maturity for purposes of clinical management is delineated in Chapter 3.

Statisticians making a determination of the status of a neonate, namely preterm or term, should define preterm as less than 259 days and term as 259 to less than 294 days in order to ensure comparable calculations with the medical community. Statisticians, by formula, subtract the date of the first day of the last menstrual period from the date of birth, whereas physicians include the first day, thus accounting for the difference.

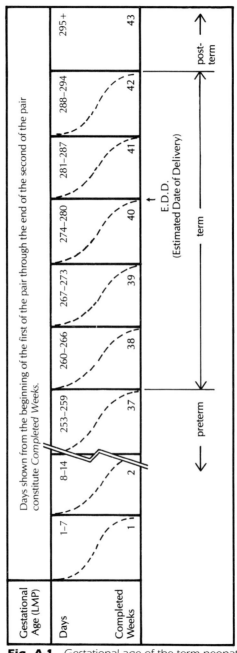

Fig. A-1. Gestational age of the term neonate.

Infant Death

Any death at any time from birth up to, but not including, 1 year of age (364 days, 23 hours, 59 minutes from the moment of birth).

Maternal Death*

The death of a woman from any cause related to or aggravated by pregnancy or its management (regardless of duration or site of pregnancy), but not from accidental or incidental causes.

Direct Obstetric Death. The death of a woman resulting from obstetric complications of pregnancy, labor, or the puerperium; from interventions, omissions, or treatment; or from a chain of events resulting from any of these.

Indirect Obstetric Death. The death of a woman resulting from a previously existing disease or a disease that developed during pregnancy, labor, or the puerperium that was not due to direct obstetric causes, although the physiologic effects of pregnancy were partially responsible for the death.

Induced Termination of Pregnancy

The purposeful interruption of an intrauterine pregnancy with the intention other than to produce a liveborn infant, and which does not result in a live birth. This definition excludes management of prolonged retention of products of conception following fetal death.

Statistical Tabulations

Statistical tabulations for vital events related to pregnancy provide the medical and statistical community with valuable information on reproductive health, as well as generating data on trends apparent in this country and worldwide. This information often is disaggregated and used to examine specific events over time or within selected geographic locations. In informing the public about health issues, media sources often

---

*Death occurring to a woman during pregnancy or after its termination from causes *not* related to the pregnancy nor to its complications or management is *not* to be considered a maternal death. Nonmaternal deaths may result from accidental causes (eg, auto accident or gunshot wound) or incidental causes (eg, concurrent malignancy).

report various statistical measures. Heightened public interest in health related issues, makes it essential that the medical community understand and have the capacity to interpret these statistics.

The following explanations of statistical tabulations provide the reader with a better understanding of measures used for events related to reproduction.

Rate is a measure of the frequency of some event in relation to a unit of population during a specified time period such as a year; events in the numerator of the rate occur to individuals in the denominator. Rates express the risk of the event in the specified population during a particular time. Rates are generally expressed as units of population in the denominator (per 1,000, per 100,000, etc.). For example, the 1982 teenaged birth rate was 52.9 live births per 1,000 women 15–19 years of age.

Ratios, on the other hand, express a *relationship* of one element to a *different* element (where the numerator is not necessarily a subset of the denominator). A ratio is generally expressed per 1,000 of the denominator element. For example, the sex ratio of live births for 1982 was 1,051 males per 1,000 females.

In the formulae that follow, "period" refers to a calendar year.

Live Birth Measures

These measures are designed to show the rate at which childbearing is occurring in the population. The crude birth rate, which relates the total number of births to the total population, gives an indication of the impact of fertility on population growth. The general fertility rate is a more specific measure of fertility since it relates the number of births to the population at risk, women in the childbearing ages (assumed to be ages 15–44 years). An even more specific set of rates, the age-specific birth rates, relates the number of births to women of a specific ages directly to the total number of women in that age group. Formulae for these measures are shown below.

$$\text{Crude Birth Rate} = \frac{\text{Number of live births to women of all ages during a calendar year} \times 1,000}{\text{Total estimated mid-year population}}$$

$$\text{General Fertility Rate} = \frac{\text{Number of live births to women of all ages during a calendar year} \times 1,000}{\text{Estimated mid-year population of women 15–44 years of age}}$$

$$\text{General Pregnancy Rate} = \frac{\text{Number of live births} + \text{number of fetal deaths} + \text{number of induced terminations of pregnancy during a calendar year} \times 1{,}000}{\text{Estimated mid-year population of women 15–44 years of age}}$$

$$\text{Age-Specific Birth Rate} = \frac{\text{Number of live births to women in a specific age group during a calendar year} \times 1{,}000}{\text{Estimated mid-year population of women in the same age group}}$$

Total Fertility Rate = The sum of age-specific birth rates of women at each age group 10–14 through 45–49. Since 5-year age groups are used, the sum is multiplied by 5. This rate can also be computed by using single years of age.

Because the birth weight of the infant is included on the birth certificate, it is possible to tabulate and focus an analysis on selected groups of live births, for example, those weighing 500 g or more.

Births can be tabulated by where they occur. Thus, they can be shown by place of occurrence, by place of residence, and by kind of setting of delivery such as at a hospital or at home. Most vital statistics tabulations are routinely tabulated by place of residence of the mother but they could be tabulated on another basis as well. What is essential, however, is that the classification be the same for all events under consideration for a specific measure.

Fetal Mortality Measures

The population at risk for fetal mortality is the number of live births plus the number of fetal deaths in a year. Alternatively, the number of live births alone is sometimes used as the population at risk. Fetal death indices indicate the likelihood that pregnancies in a population group would result in fetal death.

It is recognized that most states report fetal deaths based upon gestational age. However, birth weight can be more accurately measured than gestational age. Therefore, minimum reporting requirements of fetal deaths based upon and labeled as to specific birth weight rather than gestational age are recommended for adoption by states (see "Fetal Death" under "Reporting Requirements/Recommendations"). In addition, *statistical tabulations* of fetal deaths should include, at a minimum, fetal deaths of 500 g or more.

$$\text{Fetal Death Rate} = \frac{\begin{array}{c}\text{Number of fetal deaths}\\ \text{(of \_\_\_ weight or more)}\\ \text{during a period} \times 1{,}000\end{array}}{\begin{array}{c}\text{Number of fetal deaths}\\ \text{(of \_\_\_ weight or more)} +\\ \text{number of live births}\\ \text{during the same period}\end{array}}$$

$$\text{Fetal Death Ratio} = \frac{\begin{array}{c}\text{Number of fetal deaths}\\ \text{(of \_\_\_ weight or more)}\\ \text{during a period} \times 1{,}000\end{array}}{\begin{array}{c}\text{Number of live births}\\ \text{during the same period}\end{array}}$$

It is recognized that states will not be able to translate data from gestational age to weight immediately, and, for comparative purposes, it may be desirable to know fetal death rates for varying gestational time periods. Therefore, the collection of both weight and gestational age is recommended to allow for these comparisons. When calculating fetal death rates based upon gestational age, the number of weeks or more of stated or presumed gestation can be substituted for weight in the above formulae.

Perinatal Mortality Measures

These indices combine fetal deaths and live births which survive only briefly (up to a few days or weeks) on the assumption that similar factors are associated with these losses. The population at risk is the total number of live births plus fetal deaths, or alternatively, the number of live births. Perinatal mortality indices can vary as to age of the fetus and the infant that is included in the particular tabulation. However, the concept itself cuts across all the calculations.

It is recommended that perinatal mortality measures be based upon and labeled as to specific weight rather than gestational age (see "Reporting Requirements/Recommendations").

$$\text{Perinatal Mortality Rate} = \frac{\begin{array}{c}\text{Number of infant deaths of less}\\ \text{than \_ \_ \_ days + number of fetal deaths}\\ \text{(with stated or presumed weight}\\ \text{of \_ \_ \_ or more) during a period} \times 1{,}000\end{array}}{\begin{array}{c}\text{Number of live births + number of}\\ \text{fetal deaths (with stated or}\\ \text{presumed weight of \_ \_ \_ or more)}\\ \text{during the same period}\end{array}}$$

$$\text{Perinatal Mortality Ratio} = \frac{\begin{array}{c}\text{Number of infant deaths of less}\\ \text{than \_ \_ \_ days + number of fetal deaths}\\ \text{(with stated or presumed weight}\\ \text{of \_ \_ \_ or more) during a period} \times 1{,}000\end{array}}{\begin{array}{c}\text{Number of live births}\\ \text{during the same period}\end{array}}$$

It is recognized that states will not be able to translate data from gestational age to weight immediately, and, for purposes of comparability, knowledge of gestational age (based on last menstrual period) may be required and should be collected. When calculating perinatal death rates based upon gestational age, the number of weeks of a stated or presumed gestational age can be substituted for weight in the above formulae. When comparisons are desired based upon gestational age, the generally accepted breakdown is as follows: Perinatal Period I includes infant deaths of less than 7 days and fetal deaths with a stated or presumed period of gestation of 28 weeks or more; Perinatal Period II includes infant deaths of less than 28 days and fetal deaths with a stated or presumed period of gestation of 20 weeks or more; Perinatal Period III includes infant deaths of less than 7 days and fetal deaths with a stated or presumed gestation of 20 weeks or more (Fig. A-2).

Perinatal measures can be specific for race and other characteristics. Perinatal events can be tabulated by where they occur. Thus, they can be shown by place of occurrence, by place of residence and by place of delivery such as at a hospital or home. Most vital statistics tabulations are routinely tabulated by place of residence of the mother but they could be tabulated by place of occurrence. What is essential, however, is that the classification be the same for all events under consideration for a specific measure.

Infant Mortality Measures

Indices of infant mortality are designed to show the likelihood that live births with certain characteristics will survive the first year of life, or,

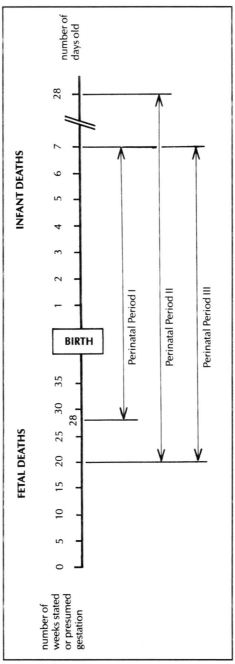

Fig. A-2. Perinatal periods.

conversely, will die during the first year of life. For infant mortality, the "population at risk" is approximated by live births that occur in a calendar year. One can compare the infant mortality rate of different population groups, such as between white and black infants. Interest sometimes focuses on two different periods in the first year of an infant's life: the very early period before the infant becomes 28 days old (up through 27 days, 23 hours, 59 minutes from the moment of birth), called the "neonatal period," and the later period starting at the end of the 28th day up to but not including one year of age (364 days, 23 hours, 59 minutes), called the "postneonatal period." Accordingly, two indices reflect these differences, namely, the neonatal mortality rate and the postneonatal mortality rate. The neonatal period can be broken down further for statistical tabulations as follows: Neonatal Period I is from the moment of birth through 23 hours and 59 minutes; Neonatal Period II starts at the end of the 24th hour of life through 6 days, 23 hours, and 59 minutes; Neonatal Period III starts at the end of the 7th day of life through 27 days, 23 hours, and 59 minutes (Fig. A-3).

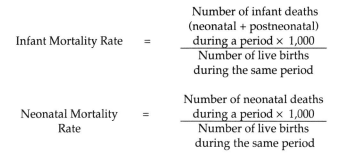

$$\text{Infant Mortality Rate} = \frac{\text{Number of infant deaths (neonatal + postneonatal) during a period} \times 1{,}000}{\text{Number of live births during the same period}}$$

$$\text{Neonatal Mortality Rate} = \frac{\text{Number of neonatal deaths during a period} \times 1{,}000}{\text{Number of live births during the same period}}$$

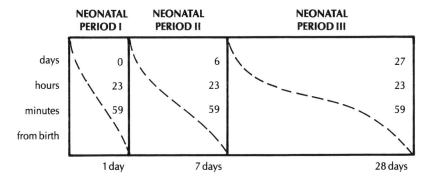

Fig. A-3. Neonatal periods.

$$\text{Postneonatal Mortality Rate} = \frac{\text{Number of postneonatal deaths during a period} \times 1{,}000}{\text{Number of live births during the same period}}$$

The denominator for the postneonatal mortality rate can also be calculated by subtracting the number of neonatal deaths from the number of live births. This denominator more accurately defines the population at risk of dying in the postneonatal period. In addition, it should be noted that infant deaths can be broken down into birth and weight categories, if desired, for comparative purposes when birth and death records are linked (see "Reporting Requirements/Recommendations").

Maternal Mortality Measures

These measures are designed to indicate the likelihood that a pregnant woman will die from complications of pregnancy, childbirth, or the puerperium. Accordingly, the population at risk is an approximation of the population of pregnant women in a year: the approximation is usually taken to be the number of live births. Maternal mortality can be examined in terms of characteristics of the woman such as age, race, and cause of death. The maternal mortality rate measures the risk of death from deliveries and complications of pregnancy, childbirth, and the puerperium.

The group exposed to risk consists of all women who have been pregnant at some time during the period. Thus, the population at risk should theoretically include all fetal deaths (reported and unreported), all induced terminations of pregnancy, and all live births. Because most states do not require the reporting of all fetal deaths and there are still a large number of states that do not require reporting of induced terminations of pregnancy, the entire population at risk can not be included in the denominator. Therefore, the total number of live births has become the generally accepted denominator. It is recommended that when complete ascertainment of the denominator (that is, the number of pregnant women) is achieved, that a modified maternal mortality rate be defined, in addition to the traditional rate.

The rate is most frequently expressed per 100,000 live births, as follows:

$$\text{Maternal Mortality Rate} = \frac{\text{Number of deaths attributed to maternal conditions during a period} \times 100{,}000}{\text{Number of live births during the same period}}$$

Cause of death rates for specified maternal causes are computed by restricting the numerator to the specified cause. The maternal mortality rates specific for race and age groups are computed by appropriately restricting both the numerator and the denominator to the specified group. Caution should be used in interpreting rates in small geographic areas; it may not be possible to generate race and age specific rates.

For statistical comparisons with the World Health Organization, it is recommended that two tabulations of statistics be prepared: 1) maternal deaths within 42 days of the end of pregnancy (WHO), and 2) with no time limitation for comparison within the United States.

Induced Termination of Pregnancy Measures

These measures parallel those of fetal deaths, but they refer to "induced" events. The population at risk for induced termination of pregnancy is taken to be live births in a year, which is used as a surrogate measure of pregnancies. Because this is not actually the total population at risk, this measure is generally considered a ratio.

$$\text{Induced Termination of Pregnancy Ratio I} = \frac{\text{Number of induced terminations occurring during a period} \times 1{,}000}{\text{Number of live births occurring during the same period}}$$

Another measure (Induced Termination of Pregnancy Ratio II) is one which, by also including an estimate of pregnancies which do not result in live births, more closely approximates the population at risk.

$$\text{Induced Termination of Pregnancy Ratio II} = \frac{\text{Number of induced terminations occurring during a period} \times 1{,}000}{\substack{\text{Number of induced terminations} \\ \text{of pregnancies} + \text{live births} + \\ \text{reported fetal deaths} \\ \text{during the same period}}}$$

Still a third measure is a rate which provides information on the *probability* that women of a certain age or race will have an induced termination of pregnancy.

$$\text{Induced Termination of Pregnancy Rate} = \frac{\text{Number of induced terminations occurring during a period} \times 1{,}000}{\text{Female population age 15–44 years}}$$

Sometimes induced termination indices are specific for certain characteristics of the woman: that is, they can refer to women of particular age or race groups.

Reporting Requirements/Recommendations

Reporting requirements for vital events related to reproductive health enable the collection of data essential to the calculation of statistical tabulations which look at trends and changes at the local, state, and national levels. The data which are used in statistical tabulations may only be a portion of those which are collected, due to the need for consistency in a tabulation, and the variations in reporting requirements from state to state. For instance, while a few states require that all fetal deaths, regardless of length of gestation, be reported, statistical tabulations of fetal death rates by the National Center for Health Statistics (NCHS) only utilize fetal deaths of 20 weeks or more gestation.

Live Birth

It is generally recognized that all states report all live births as defined in the definitions section of this document. It is recommended that all live births be reported regardless of birth weight, length of gestation, or survival time.

Fetal Death

Reporting requirements for fetal deaths now vary from state to state. At present, most states require reporting of fetal deaths by gestational age. It is generally recognized that birth weight can be more accurately measured than gestational age.

It must be emphasized that a specific birth weight criterion for reporting of fetal deaths does not imply a point of viability and should be chosen instead for its feasibility in collecting useful data.

Current statistical tabulations of fetal deaths, include, at a minimum, fetal deaths of 500 grams or more. Furthermore, all but three states now require either reporting of all fetal deaths or reporting of some fetal deaths below 500 grams, for example, those which fall below 500 grams because of the variation in birth weights at a given required gestational age such as 20 weeks. Therefore, it is recommended that

- Statistical tabulations for comparisons of perinatal mortality rates within the United States exclude fetal deaths of less than 500 g.

- Each state adopt a specific birth weight criterion for reporting of fetal deaths which will result in continued collection of data on as close as possible to 100% of the population of fetal deaths currently reported in that state. When birth weight is unknown, an estimate of gestation age should be utilized to determine whether or not this event is required to be reported.
- All state fetal death report forms include birth weight and gestational age.

Perinatal Mortality

Perinatal mortality indices generally combine fetal deaths and live births which survive only briefly (up to a few days or weeks). Since reporting requirements on fetal deaths vary from state to state, perinatal mortality reporting will also vary (see previous section on Perinatal Periods).

As with fetal deaths, it is recommended that perinatal mortality be weight specific. However, for purposes of comparability, knowledge of gestational age (based on last menstrual period) should be collected.

Infant Mortality

All states require that all infant deaths (neonatal plus postneonatal) as defined in the definitions section of this document be reported.

Infant deaths by birth weight are not routinely available for the United States as a whole since birth weight information is not collected on the death certificate. However, since birth weight is reported on the birth certificate, by linking together the birth certificate and the death certificate for the same infant, it is possible to obtain information on infant deaths by birth weight. At the present time, most states link birth and death certificates. It is recommended that this be encouraged to create a national data base for infant mortality by birth weight.

In addition, it is recommended that infant death reports include the exact interval from birth rather than categories such as neonatal or postneonatal. This too, will allow for more specific age-related death analyses.

Maternal Mortality

Every state is required to report all maternal deaths. Since annual deaths attributed to maternal mortality only approximate 300, emphasis must be placed on in-depth investigations. Case-finding, together with individual review and analysis of risk factors contributing to maternal deaths, is of the highest importance. Collection of data regarding these rare events is critical, when combined, as it should be, with educational review by those closest to the case, usually the obstetrician–gynecologists in the hospital and the surrounding region. Such analysis can yield clinical information about risk factors associated, for example, with detection and treatment of ectopic pregnancies, or with anesthesia. This clinical information can then be gathered and exchanged to help practitioners identify risk factors which contribute to maternal death and associated conditions.

Induced Termination of Pregnancy

The United States has no national system for reporting induced terminations of pregnancy. State health departments vary greatly in their approaches to the compilation of these data from compiling no data to: 1) periodically requesting hospitals, clinics and/or physicians performing the procedures to voluntarily report total number of procedures performed; 2) requiring (by legislative or regulatory authority) hospitals, clinics and/or physicians to periodically report aggregate level data on number or number and characteristics of procedures; or, 3) requiring (by legal or regulatory authority) hospitals, clinics, and/or physicians to periodically report individual level data on each procedure performed.

Since 1969, the Division of Reproductive Health (DRH), Centers for Disease Control (CDC), has published an annual Abortion Surveillance Report based upon data provided from state health departments, when available, and from data voluntarily provided to CDC from hospitals and clinics in states with no data available from health departments. In addition to information on the number and characteristics of induced terminations of pregnancy, the Abortion Surveillance Report contains information from CDC's abortion mortality surveillance, which was begun with the cooperation of state health departments in 1972. Investigation and review of each related death by DRH epidemiologists result in improved detailed nosological identification of abortion mortality by type of risk.*

Since 1977, the National Center for Health Statistics has analyzed the induced terminations of pregnancy occurring in up to 13 states in which individual reports of induced terminations are submitted to state vital

---

*The CDC Abortion Surveillance Report includes information on events categorized by CDC as abortions (legal, illegal, and spontaneous). While this terminology preexisted the recommendations in this paper and is at variance with the definition herein, it has been commonly used and understood to include induced termination of pregnancy.

registration offices. In addition, the Alan Guttmacher Institute, a private organization, publishes information on induced terminations that it obtains from a nationwide survey of induced termination providers.

Collecting information on the number of induced terminations of pregnancy, the characteristics of women having such procedures, and the number and characteristics of all deaths related to induced termination of pregnancy would be extremely valuable in identifying and evaluating risk factors for specific population groups and for the public in general. By gathering these data, studies could be instituted with practitioners. Knowing the outcomes could further the body of knowledge and ultimately reduce the risks.

Therefore, we urge state health departments that compile statistics on induced terminations of pregnancy to evaluate and improve the quality of their data. Furthermore, we urge state health departments that do not compile such statistics to explore mechanisms for initiating their collection.

Current Reporting Requirements

The following general fetal death reporting requirements, as of March 1991, should be brought into conformity with the recommendations in this report:

20 weeks or more gestation

Alabama	Iowa	Oklahoma
Alaska	Maryland*	Oregon*
Arizona*	Minnesota	Texas
California	Montana	Utah
Connecticut	Nebraska	Vermont*
Delaware	Nevada	Washington
Florida	New Jersey	West Virginia
Guam	North Carolina	Wyoming
Illinois	North Dakota	
Indiana	Ohio	

20 weeks or more gestation or birth weight of 500 g or more

District of Columbia

---

*Specific modifiers apply

20 weeks or more gestation or birth weight of 350 g or more

Idaho	Massachusetts	New Hampshire
Kentucky	Mississippi	South Carolina
Louisiana	Missouri	Wisconsin

Birth weight in excess of 350 g

Kansas

20 weeks or more gestation or birth weight of 400 g or more

Michigan

Birth weight of 500 g or more

New Mexico
South Dakota
Tennessee*

5 months or more gestation

Puerto Rico

16 weeks or more gestation

Pennsylvania

All products of human conception

American Samoa	Maine	Rhode Island
Arkansas	New York City	Virginia
Colorado	New York State	Virgin Islands
Georgia	Northern Mariana	
Hawaii	Islands	

---

*Specific modifiers apply

APPENDIX G

Resources from ACOG and AAP

The ACOG Technical Bulletin Series of the American College of Obstetricians and Gynecologists is designed to provide practicing physicians with the latest proven techniques of clinical practice. ACOG Committee Opinions are intended to provide timely information on controversial issues, ethical concerns, and emerging approaches to clinical management. Subscriptions and complete sets of all Technical Bulletins or Committee Opinions in print, with or without a three-ring binder, are available for sale. Contact the ACOG Resource Center for a current list and order forms for both series. (Because individual Technical Bulletins and Committee Opinions are withdrawn from and added to the series, some of the titles listed here may no longer be current.)

ACOG Technical Bulletins

Number	Title	Date
59	Management of Gestational Trophoblastic Neoplasia	December 1980
62	Rubella: A Clinical Update	July 1981
84	Teratology	February 1985
86	Grief Related to Perinatal Death	April 1985
87	Women and Exercise	September 1985
91	Management of Preeclampsia	March 1986
92	Management of Diabetes Mellitus in Pregnancy	May 1986
95	Management of Breech Presentation	August 1986
96	Drug Abuse and Pregnancy	September 1986
98	Diagnosis and Management of Fetal Death	November 1986
107	Antepartum Fetal Surveillance	August 1987
108	Antenatal Diagnosis of Genetic Disorders	September 1987
112	Obstetric Anesthesia and Analgesia	January 1988
114	Perinatal Viral and Parasitic Infections	March 1988
115	Premature Rupture of Membranes	April 1988
116	Ultrasound in Pregnancy	May 1988
117	Antimicrobial Therapy for Obstetric Patients	June 1988
121	Invasive Hemodynamic Monitoring in Obstetrics and Gynecology	October 1988

Number	Title	Date
122	Perinatal Herpes Simplex Virus Infections	November 1988
123	Human Immune Deficiency Virus Infections	December 1988
124	The Battered Woman	January 1989
127	Assessment of Fetal and Newborn Acid–Base Status	April 1989
130	Postterm Pregnancy	July 1989
131	Multiple Gestation	August 1989
132	Intrapartum Fetal Heart Rate Monitoring	September 1989
133	Preterm Labor	October 1989
136	Ethical Decision-Making in Obstetrics and Gynecology	November 1989
137	Dystocia	December 1989
143	Diagnosis and Management of Postpartum Hemorrhage	July 1990
145	The Adolescent Obstetric–Gynecologic Patient	September 1990
147	Prevention of D Isoimmunization	October 1990
148	Management of Isoimmunization in Pregnancy	October 1990
151	Automobile Passenger Restraints for Children and Pregnant Women	January 1991
152	Operative Vaginal Delivery	February 1991
154	Alpha-Fetoprotein	April 1991
157	Induction and Augmentation of Labor	July 1991
159	Fetal Macrosomia	September 1991
160	Immunization During Pregnancy	October 1991
161	Trauma During Pregnancy	November 1991

ACOG Committee Opinions

Number	Title	Date
49	Use and Misuse of the Apgar Score *Committee on Obstetrics: Maternal and Fetal Medicine (ACOG) and Committee on Fetus and Newborn (AAP)*	November 1986 (Reaffirmed 1991)
50	Postpartum Tubal Sterilization: Appropriate Timing of Surgery After Vaginal Delivery *Committee on Obstetrics: Maternal and Fetal Medicine*	February 1987 (Reaffirmed 1989)
52	Vitamin A Supplementation During Pregnancy *Committee on Obstetrics: Maternal and Fetal Medicine*	July 1987 (Reaffirmed 1991)

55	Patient Choice: Maternal–Fetal Conflict *Committee on Ethics*	October 1987
58	Alcohol and Pregnancy *Committee on Obstetrics: Maternal and Fetal Medicine*	October 1987 (Reaffirmed 1989)
61	Ethical Issues in Pregnancy Counseling *Committee on Ethics*	March 1988
62	Contraceptives and Congenital Anomalies *Committee on Gynecologic Practice*	September 1988 (Reaffirmed 1990)
64	Guidelines for Vaginal Delivery After a Previous Cesarean Birth *Committee on Obstetrics: Maternal and Fetal Medicine*	October 1988 (Reaffirmed 1991)
69	Chorionic Villus Sampling *Committee on Obstetrics: Maternal and Fetal Medicine*	November 1989 (Reaffirmed 1991)
71	Obstetric Forceps *Committee on Obstetrics: Maternal and Fetal Medicine*	August 1989 (Reaffirmed 1991)
74	Strategies to Prevent Prematurity: Home Uterine Activity Monitoring *Committee on Obstetrics: Maternal and Fetal Medicine*	November 1989 (Reaffirmed 1991)
76	Maternal Serum Alpha-Fetoprotein *Committee on Obstetrics: Maternal and Fetal Medicine*	December 1989 (Reaffirmed 1991)
79	Scope of Services for Uncomplicated Obstetric Care *Committee on Obstetrics: Maternal and Fetal Medicine*	January 1990 (Reaffirmed 1991)
81	Cocaine Abuse: Implications for Pregnancy *Committee on Obstetrics: Maternal and Fetal Medicine*	March 1990
83	Management of Labor and Delivery for Patients with Spinal Cord Injury *Committee on Obstetrics: Maternal and Fetal Medicine*	May 1990
85	HIV Infection: Physicians' Responsibilities *Committee on Ethics*	September 1990
87	Deception *Committee on Ethics*	November 1990
88	Ethical Issues in Surrogate Motherhood *Committee on Ethics*	November 1990

Number	Title	Date
91	Umbilical Cord Blood Acid–Base Sampling *Committee on Obstetrics: Maternal and Fetal Medicine*	February 1991
92	Statement on Surgical Assistants *Committee on Gynecologic Practice; Committee on Obstetrics: Maternal and Fetal Medicine*	March 1991
93	Screening for Tay-Sachs Disease *Committee on Obstetrics: Maternal and Fetal Medicine*	March 1991
94	Multifetal Pregnancy Reduction and Selective Fetal Termination *Committee on Ethics*	April 1991
96	Ultrasound Imaging in Pregnancy *Committee on Obstetrics: Maternal and Fetal Medicine*	August 1991
97	Voluntary Testing for Human Immunodeficiency Virus *Committee on Obstetrics: Maternal and Fetal Medicine*	September 1991
98	Fetal Maturity Assessment Prior to Elective Repeat Cesarean Delivery *Committee on Obstetrics: Maternal and Fetal Medicine*	September 1991
99	Lyme Disease During Pregnancy *Committee on Obstetrics: Maternal and Fetal Medicine*	November 1991
101	Current Status of Cystic Fibrosis Carrier Screening *Committee on Obstetrics: Maternal and Fetal Medicine*	November 1991
102	Placental Pathology *Committee on Obstetrics: Maternal and Fetal Medicine*	December 1991

AAP Committee Statements/Publications

Copies of the following documents are available through the American Academy of Pediatrics Publications Department, 141 Northwest Point Blvd., PO Box 927, Oak Grove Village, IL 60009-0927; (708) 228-5005.

Title	Date
Aluminum Toxicity in Infants and Children *Committee on Nutrition*	December 1986
Commentary on Parenteral Nutrition *Committee on Nutrition*	April 1983 (Reaffirmed 1987)
Dexamethasone Therapy for Bacterial Meningitis in Infants and Children *Committee on Infectious Diseases*	July 1990
Drug-Exposed Infants *Committee on Substance-Abuse*	October 1990
Emergency Drug Doses for Infants and Children *Committee on Drugs*	March 1988
Emergency Drug Doses for Infants and Children and Naloxone Use in Newborns: Clarification *Committee on Drugs*	May 1989
Encouraging Breast-Feeding *Committee on Nutrition*	March 1980 (Reaffirmed 1991)
Fetal Research *Council on Pediatric Research*	September 1984
Fetal Therapy: Ethical Considerations *Committee on Bioethics*	June 1988
Fluoride Supplementation *Committee on Nutrition*	May 1986 (Reaffirmed 1989)
Follow-up on Weaning Formulas *Committee on Nutrition*	June 1989
Guidelines for Infant Bioethics Committees *Committee on Bioethics*	August 1984 (Reaffirmed 1987)
Guidelines for the Elective Use of Conscious Sedation, Deep Sedation, and General Anesthesia in Pediatric Patients *Committee on Drugs*	May 1986 (Under revision)
High-Risk Newborn Care *Committee on Practice and Ambulatory Medicine; Committee on Fetus and Newborn*	July 1985 (Reaffirmed 1991)

Title	Date
Home Phototherapy *Committee on Fetus and Newborn*	July 1985 (Reaffirmed 1991)
Hypoallergenic Infant Formulas *Committee on Nutrition*	June 1989
Imitation and Substitute Milks *Committee on Nutrition*	June 1984 (Reaffirmed 1991)
Infant Methemoglobinemia: The Role of Dietary Nitrate *Committee on Nutrition*	September 1970 (Reaffirmed 1991)
Infant Radiant Warmers *Committee on Environmental Hazards*	January 1978 (Reaffirmed 1986)
Infants and Children with Acquired Immunodeficiency Syndrome: Placement in Adoption and Foster Care *Task Force on Pediatric AIDS*	April 1989 (Under revision)
Iron-Fortified Infant Formulas *Committee on Nutrition*	December 1989
Iron Supplementation for Infants *Committee on Nutrition*	November 1976 (Reaffirmed 1987)
Issues in Newborn Screening *Committee on Genetics*	(Approved for publication)
Manpower Needs in Neonatal Pediatrics *Committee on Fetus and Newborn*	July 1985 (Reaffirmed 1990)
Maternal Phenylketonuria *Committee on Genetics*	(Approved for publication)
Maternal Serum α-Fetoprotein Screening *Committee on Genetics*	(Approved for publication)
Naloxone Dosage and Route of Administration for Infants and Children: Addendum to Emergency Drug Doses for Infants and Children *Committee on Drugs*	September 1990
Naloxone Use in Newborns *Committee on Drugs*	March 1980 (Reaffirmed 1990)
Neonatal Anesthesia *Committee on Fetus and Newborn; Committee on Drugs; Section on Anesthesiology; Section on Surgery*	September 1987 (Reaffirmed 1990)

Title	Date
Neonatal Anesthesia *Committee on Fetus and Newborn; Committee on Drugs; Section on Anesthesiology; Section on Surgery*	September 1987 (Reaffirmed 1990)
Neonatal Drug Withdrawal *Committee on Drugs*	December 1983 (Reaffirmed 1990)
Neonatal Nurse Clinicians *Committee on Fetus and Newborn*	December 1982 (Under revision)
Newborn Screening Fact Sheets *Committee on Genetics*	March 1989
Newborn Screening for Congenital Hypothyroidism *Committee on Genetics*	November 1987 (Under revision)
Noise Pollution *Committee on Environmental Hazards*	November 1986 (Reaffirmed 1991)
Nutrition and Lactation *Committee on Nutrition*	September 1981 (Reaffirmed 1987)
Nutritional Needs of Low Birthweight Infants *Committee on Nutrition*	May 1985 (Reaffirmed 1987)
Parvovirus, Erythema Infectiosum and Pregnancy *Committee on Infectious Diseases*	January 1990
Pediatric Guidelines for Infection Control of HIV (AIDS) in Hospitals, Medical Offices, Schools, and Other Settings *Task Force on Pediatric AIDS*	November 1988
Pediatrician's Responsibility for Infant Nutrition *AAP Executive Board*	October 1986
Perinatal HIV Infection (AIDS) *Task Force on Pediatric AIDS*	December 1988
Prenatal Diagnosis for Pediatricians *Committee on Genetics*	October 1989
The Prenatal Visit *Committee on Psychosocial Aspects of Child and Family Health*	April 1984
Promotion of Breast-Feeding *AAP Task Force*	May 1982
Recommendations on Extracorporeal Membrane Oxygenation *Committee on Fetus and Newborn*	April 1990

Title	Date
Report of the Committee on Infectious Diseases *Committee on Infectious Diseases*	1991
Reimbursement for Medical Foods for Inborn Errors of Amino Acid Metabolism *Committee on Nutrition*	April 1979 (Reaffirmed 1987)
Report of the Task Force on Circumcision *Task Force on Circumcision*	August 1989
Ribavirin Therapy of Respiratory Syncytial Virus *Committee on Infectious Diseases*	March 1987
Safe Transportation of Newborns Discharged from the Hospital *Committee on Injury and Poison Prevention*	September 1990
Safe Transportation of Premature Infants *Committee on Injury and Poison Prevention; Committee on Fetus and Newborn*	January 1991
Soy-Protein Formulas: Use in Infant Feeding *Committee on Nutrition*	September 1983 (Reaffirmed 1991)
Surfactant Replacement Therapy for Respiratory Distress Syndrome *Committee on Fetus and Newborn*	June 1991
Transfer of Drugs and Other Chemicals into Human Milk *Committee on Drugs*	November 1989
Treatment of Bacterial Meningitis *Committee on Infectious Diseases*	June 1988
Treatment of Congenital Hypothyroidism *Committee on Drugs*	September 1978 (Under revision)
Treatment of Critically Ill Newborns *Committee on Bioethics*	October 1983 (Reaffirmed 1987)
Use and Abuse of the Apgar Score *Committee on Fetus and Newborn*	December 1986 (Reaffirmed 1990)
Use of Whole Cow's Milk in Infancy *Committee on Nutrition*	August 1983 (Under revision)
Valproate Teratogenicity *Committee on Drugs*	June 1983 (Reaffirmed 1990)
WIC Program *AAP Executive Board*	June 1988

INDEX

Doxycycline, for chlamydial infection, 137
Draining lesions, in neonate, isolation procedures for, 158–159
Dress codes, for hospital personnel, 148–149
Drug abuse. See Substance abuse
Drug-exposed infants, 224–230
    health policy issues raised by, 226–227
    pediatric implications of, 225–226
Drugs, for resuscitation of neonate, 89
DTP. See Diphtheria, tetanus, and pertussis vaccine

Early intervention, 114–115
Echovirus infection, 159
EDD. See Estimated date of delivery
Education
    in-service and continuing education, 10–11
    parent, postpartum, 104–105
    perinatal outreach programs, 11–12
Electrical outlets and electrical equipment, for newborn care areas, 32
Emergency medical condition
    special determination of, for pregnant women, 245–246
    statutory definition of, 245
Emotional lability, postpartum, 112
Endometritis
    and breast-feeding, 184
    chlamydial, 137
    group A streptococcal, isolation procedures for, 156
    incidence of, 151
    management of, 151–52
    postcesarean, 151–152
    signs and symptoms of, 151
Enterovirus infection, of neonate, 142
Environmental control, in infection prevention, 166–167
Epilepsy, 221–223
Epinephrine hydrochloride, in neonatal resuscitation, 89

Episiotomy
    indications for, 80
    pain after, analgesia for, 97, 98
    postpartum care with, 97
Erythema infectiosum, 128
Erythema migrans, 135
Erythroblastosis fetalis, and bilirubin toxicity, 204–206
Erythromycin
    for chlamydial infection, 137
    for Lyme disease, 137
    in prevention of chlamydial conjunctivitis, 138
    in prevention of gonococcal ophthalmia neonatorum, 94
Escherichia coli infection
    epidemic, in nursery, 162–164
    of neonate, 142
Estimated date of delivery, establishment of, 54
Ethylene oxide, in sterilization, 167–168
Evacuation policy, for perinatal care areas, 32
Exchange transfusion
    in hemolytic disease, 207
    in management of neonatal jaundice, 206, 208
External cardiac massage, in neonatal resuscitation, 87–88

Face masks, cleaning and disinfection of, 172
Failure to thrive, 113, 183
Family, participation in childbirth education programs, 51
Fertility rate
    general, 258
    total, 259
Fetal death(s)/mortality. See also Perinatal loss; Perinatal mortality
    definition of, 255
    measures of, for statistical tabulations, 259–260
    rate, 260
        age-specific, calculation of, 193
    ratio, 260